Dialysis
without
Fear

Dialysis
without
Fear

A Guide to Living Well on Dialysis
for Patients and Their Families

Daniel Offer, M.D.
Marjorie Kaiz Offer
Susan Offer Szafir

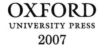

OXFORD
UNIVERSITY PRESS
2007

OXFORD

UNIVERSITY PRESS

Oxford University Press, Inc., publishes works that further
Oxford University's objective of excellence
in research, scholarship, and education.

Oxford   New York
Auckland   Cape Town   Dar es Salaam   Hong Kong   Karachi
Kuala Lumpur   Madrid   Melbourne   Mexico City   Nairobi
New Delhi   Shanghai   Taipei   Toronto

With offices in
Argentina   Austria   Brazil   Chile   Czech Republic   France   Greece
Guatemala   Hungary   Italy   Japan   Poland   Portugal   Singapore
South Korea   Switzerland   Thailand   Turkey   Ukraine   Vietnam

Published by Oxford University Press, Inc.
198 Madison Avenue, New York, New York 10016
www.oup.com

Oxford is a registered trademark of Oxford University Press

Library of Congress Cataloging-in-Publication Data
Offer, Daniel.
Dialysis without fear : a guide to living well
on dialysis for patients and their families
/ Daniel Offer, M.D., Marjorie Kaiz Offer, Susan Offer Szafir.
p. cm.   Includes bibliographical references and index.
ISBN 978-0-19-530994-2—ISBN 978-0-19-530995-9 (paper)
1. Hemodialysis—Popular works.
2. Chronic renal failure—Popular works.
I. Offer, Marjorie Kaiz.
II. Szafir, Susan Offer, 1971–
III. Title.
RC918.R4026 2007
617.4'61059—dc22   2006102678

1 3 5 7 9 8 6 4 2
Printed in the United States of America
on acid-free paper

To all those brave souls who deal with dialysis

To Ariel with love and gratitude

Contents

Preface

WHEN A NEPHROLOGIST, a doctor specializing in kidney function, tells a patient his or her kidneys have failed to the point of no return and he or she will need ongoing dialysis or a transplant to live, a barrage of questions is sure to follow. At that moment, or over the course of the next days and months, that person will certainly wonder, "What is dialysis? How does it work? Will it hurt? How will it impact my family? How will others view me? Will I be sick all the time? Will life be worth living? Will I die? Will I be able to work? To travel? To eat and drink as I please? To have sex? To parent a child?" And the list goes on.

Most dialysis patients will tell you that the initial adjustment to life on dialysis, whether they are awaiting a transplant or not, is no small undertaking. Nor is the ongoing battle of working through the fears associated with dialysis. Going on dialysis is a major life transition invariably accompanied by a watershed of emotions and uncertainties. In fact, it is debatable which is initially more profound: the emotional or the physical impact.

In the past, "end stage" renal disease appeared to be an appropriate term. As recently as the 1970s there were many hardships associated with it: a lack of dialysis machines to accommodate everyone in need, high rates of anemia, and hemodialysis sessions that could last for sixteen hours.[1] But today everyone in the United States needing dialysis can be treated. Modern medicines have significantly minimized rates of anemia. Advancements of technologies have reduced hemodialysis sessions to three to five hours in duration and have introduced alternative forms of dialysis that give patients more flexibility and control of their care. And yet, while dialysis has evolved significantly over the last several decades, negative perceptions about life on dialysis among the majority of the general population have not.

Today many persons with kidney failure are no longer definitively facing the end of their lives. Instead they are approaching a new chapter that, despite large challenges and lifestyle changes, can be fully lived and enjoyed for many years. But this reality is not often apparent to those new to dialysis, as it certainly wasn't apparent to us when we were first introduced to it. It is this reality that ultimately led us, after several years of being immersed in the world of dialysis, to decide to write this book.

And who are we? Together, we are Daniel, Margie, and Susan—the three co-authors of this book—and from this point forward will refer to ourselves as such. Respectively, we are the psychiatrist, the researcher, and the writer. We are also, respectively, the patient, the spouse, and their adult child. Working together, using each of these skills and perspectives, we were able to bring what began as a glimmer of an idea to fruition.

This idea took root a few years ago when Daniel delivered an inspirational and light-hearted keynote speech about living well on dialysis. The speech defied the stereotypical misconception that dialysis patients are invalids and became the seed of an idea for a book that we wished had existed when Daniel first encountered his kidney failure and the resulting dialysis in 1999. We thought, what if there had been a book written by a patient and family members specifically for other patients and family members? What if there had been a book that informatively, realistically, and even at times humorously laid out a road map for successfully living well on dialysis, and that covered a range of practical and personal topics from dining out to traveling to working? What if the book had been interesting, relevant, and—can you imagine—enjoyable to read? Certainly the three of us, and even others near and dear to Daniel, would have read it from cover to cover. And in doing so, our learning curve associated with adapting to dialysis would have been less steep and our initiation to this new world would have been less daunting. Alas, there was no such book, or at least none that we could find.

Today we are proud to have written such a book; however, our perspectives are not the only ones you will hear. Before putting pen to paper, we met and spoke with numerous dialysis patients and medical professionals who weighed in about what it means to live well on dialysis and about which persons do so and how. We relied on medical professionals to refer fellow patients to us. We asked doctors, nurses, and social workers to introduce us to folks who were in their eyes "living well" on dialysis. We granted anonymity to each person we met—patient or otherwise—in hopes that he or she would feel comfortable sharing intimate details and true opinions. For this reason, names, places, and other information about the identity of the individuals described in these pages have been altered. But other than that, the stories are quite real and so are the people telling them.

As you will see, this promise of anonymity worked. The people we spoke with did not pull punches; they did not attempt to stifle their opinions. Our intent was not to sugarcoat dialysis, so we included many of the honest-to-goodness opinions that we gathered, even the most negative. At the same time, we shared what we heard many others say, which was often very hopeful. Ultimately, the opinions throughout the book should be taken seriously—but remember, they are opinions. Much of dialysis is about choices, and once a patient chooses to follow a specific course of treatment, his or her healthy emotional response is to advocate the path chosen wholeheartedly. In other words, at times, you may need to take some of the very strongest of opinions that advocate this or that path with a grain of salt and to understand them in the context of a given person's particular situation.

Another point to bear in mind while reading this book: it has been written for adults dealing with dialysis. We felt that pediatric dialysis likely warranted a separate book entirely. But if you are a parent of a child coping with chronic kidney disease, you will still find much of this book to be of interest. Likewise, this book was not written specifically for people who are suffering from comorbid (i.e., co-occurring) diseases, such as cancer, when renal failure is just one symptom of the disease. Even so, there are sections of the book that will be of value to persons coping with such diseases.

In the end, the compilation of the voices and stories herein, interspersed with facts and other information about dialysis, should resonate with our readers as if they have been talking to an old friend—an old friend who has walked down an uncharted path before them, and having walked ahead can now provide readers with a map. The map highlights treacherous sand traps, prickly bushes, beautiful overlooks, and comfortable pit stops. Each road marker serves as a valuable piece of information, and collectively they provide one with a general idea of what to expect on the journey. Having a sense of what is up the road ahead will, we hope, make the journey less frightening.

Of course, we are sorry that you, our readers, have joined us on this particular road. Truthfully, it is at times a little harder to walk than certain others. But it can be traveled! More important, it can be traveled with enjoyment, and we would be honored to show you the way.

Acknowledgments

Tᴴɪꜱ ʙᴏᴏᴋ ᴡᴀꜱ a collaborative effort. We'd like to thank all the
people who contributed. Thank you to Polly Jacobson, M.D.,
and James Jacobson, M.D., for encouraging us to write this book.
Our gratitude also extends to Barbara Burgess for helping us to craft
our message, to Ivan Dee for his guidance on navigating the world of
publishing, and to Mariclaire Cloutier for opening the right doors.
We'd also like to thank several members of the National Kidney
Foundation of Illinois who shared with us their expertise, including
Willa Lang, Dorothy Zecca, Nancy Lepain, Kimberly Fowler, Carole
K. Love, and Kate O'Conner. We appreciate the time we spent talk-
ing to Domeena C. Renshaw, M.D., regarding sexuality and chronic
illness. Thanks to Frederic L. Coe, M.D. and Craig B. Langman,
M.D. for their ongoing assistance. We extend our gratitude to Sandra
Downey for her help in preparing the manuscript. Thank you to
Carolyn Brooks for reading and critiquing the book and to Kristi
Robinson for connecting us with many of the individuals we interviewed. We owe a tremendous debt of gratitude to these anonymous
individuals who spoke to us candidly about dialysis and their life experiences. Thank you to the many nephrologists, nurses, technicians,
social workers, dieticians, family members, and especially patients.
We could not have written this book without you.

On a more personal note, many thanks go to Ariel Szafir for reading and rereading this book in his second language. Thank you to Lisa
Nguyen for keeping the Szafir family afloat. Thank you to the Shabbat
group, the Fuqua women, and especially the two Virginia gals, for

their ongoing support and encouragement. We are most appreciative of our editor, Marion Osmun, who has helped us write the best book we know how and of Sarah Harrington for helping shepherd it to print. Thank you to Norman Simon, M.D., Daniel's nephrologist, who has been with us every step of the way, whether supervising Daniel's medical care or helping with each phase of this book.

Dialysis
without
Fear

One

Dialysis Misperceptions versus Realities

THE KIDNEY SPECIALIST, a nephrologist, gestures to the mounds of journals, pamphlets, and magazines that litter his office and says, "Welcome to the land of dialysis. It is a very complicated world. A person could spend a lifetime studying everything there is to know about it." As he sweeps his arm at the stacks of literature, one thing is immediately clear: dialysis isn't as simple as visiting the dentist or having your tires rotated. In fact, as you may or may not know, it is abundantly more comprehensive in scope and complex in nature.

Unfortunately, this complexity can often breed confusion, misunderstandings, and misinterpretations, which in themselves can often create undue anxiety, depression, and fear for a patient or family member who is new to dialysis. But these emotions can be minimized from the start simply by being "in the know" about the most common and detrimental misperceptions out there. And replacing these misperceptions with real perspectives and facts—about what dialysis *is* versus what it *is not*—will be an important step in dealing with this "complicated world." Let's begin by hearing one woman's views on her own experience of that world. As you read this and other accounts in this chapter, you'll find certain terminology—for example, *hemodialysis, peritoneal dialysis, access,* and so on—that may be unfamiliar to you. These terms will be explained in subsequent chapters and are also briefly defined in the book's glossary. For now, we simply want to introduce you to the overall experience of dialysis—the questions, the challenges, the adjustments—that some veterans of the treatment have encountered and successfully mastered.

Donna's Story, a Patient's Perspective

Entering the dialysis clinic, Susan asks to speak with Donna and is directed to a heavyset African American woman seated at the end of the first row of chairs. Despite the tubes full of blood flowing from her left arm, Donna greets Susan with a twinkle in her eye and a warm smile. Susan quickly learns that Donna is fifty-six years old and has been on hemodialysis for almost four years. Diagnosed at age twenty-two with diabetes, Donna's reliance on dialysis some thirty years later is attributed to this disease, which runs in her family. Over those thirty years she heard the word dialysis but didn't know exactly what it was, and she says, "I really didn't expect it to happen to me." Even when she was entered into an experimental drug study that tracked the increasing failure of her kidneys over three years, she recalls she still "didn't take it seriously. I didn't know what dialysis was or what kidney failure was."

Eventually her primary care doctor referred her to a nephrologist who broke the news to her; her kidneys were failing. She saw the kidney specialist quite a few times before going on dialysis. The doctor continuously tested her blood and waited for the chemical indicators of kidney failure to elevate to the point that she was eligible for the treatment. During this time the nephrologist gave her educational videos to watch, which she did, but according to Donna, "It still took being here and sitting in this chair for me to finally understand what was going on."

Donna describes her initiation to dialysis as a difficult one. "When I first started dialysis I felt restricted of course. I felt like I was going to die. I couldn't imagine those needles in my arm. I thought it was a desperate situation. Dialysis was devastating to me." Susan asks Donna if she thought about giving up. "Well, I guess I could have thought about giving up, but I have a family. They didn't think about me giving up, so it wasn't an option for me." Now Donna says she feels differently about dialysis. She is much more comfortable with the situation, but there is a lot she has learned over her four years of treatment that has increased her comfort.

Her family's comfort level has improved as well. Initially her two grown sons and her husband were just as scared as she was. She figures, "They probably thought it was a death sentence for me." Her husband Joe, whom she has been married to for thirty-six years, initially came with her to every treatment. Now he still makes a point to stop by almost every session and brings her lunch when he can. His devotion to his wife has continued, although Donna says, "He seems not to be as concerned as he was in the beginning."

Susan asks Donna a number of questions about the four years she has spent on dialysis and what she would like to pass along to patients and their families new to the treatment:

What do you wish someone had told you when you first started dialysis?

"First of all, I know a lot of people who are diabetic and are heading toward dialysis. You try to tell them about dialysis but they don't listen. They don't seem to understand the seriousness of this. It is like trying to talk to a smoker who refuses to quit.

"I wish someone had told me that dialysis was permanent. Instead they told me that I had a choice between peritoneal dialysis and hemodialysis. It was very discouraging to find out later that I really didn't have a choice because of my weight. The same was true for a transplant. It was very disappointing to be given false hope. I'm certain if I could lose the weight they would put me on a transplant list. Unfortunately, the weight loss is something I've never been able to do. They recommended gastric bypass surgery for me. But I thought the procedure was too risky, as did my husband and other family members, so I gave up on that idea. Every individual's personal health situation is different. You need to ask a lot of questions and evaluate what really is feasible for you.

"I want to be realistic about dialysis—I want to let people know that it can be awful—but I also want people to know they can do it. Dialysis is not so horrible; it is just the sitting here so long, the monotony, what happens to you on these machines, the restrictions. If you don't follow the restrictions you can really suffer. Dialysis doesn't hurt. It is just boring as hell. Best thing to do is accept dialysis and then leave it. Leave it where it is."

What advice would you give to someone who is new to dialysis?

"Be patient. Learn as much about this machine as you can. Learn how to cope with being here and the illness that you have. Realize that you have to do this to survive. Make sure that you like the personnel, and they are knowledgeable about what is going on. Always be alert and aware of your surroundings as well as your care. It is important for people to explain to you what they are doing while they are doing it. It is important for people to treat you with respect. If you aren't finding this, if you don't feel like you see the doctor enough, if no one asks you how you are feeling, then something is wrong. If something is not right, if you are not happy with your clinic or the technicians speak up or change your situation. At our clinic we have a patient advocacy committee, which is helpful. If we do have problems, we can bring them up without fear of retaliation."

Specifically, Donna's comfort level improved dramatically when she changed dialysis clinics after a year of treatment. At her first clinic, as she became more knowledgeable about what the technicians should know, she became increasingly dissatisfied. She did not like, for example, how the patients who were very elderly or less alert were cared for. On the other hand, she really liked her doctor and was hesitant to change clinics. She gave the clinic a year, but ultimately decided the patients there were not treated with the dignity and respect they deserved. She felt it was up to her to improve her situation, and so not only did she change to a new clinic, but she also became an active participant on its patient advocacy committee.

Are there any tricks you've learned that help you manage your diet and your liquid intake?

"I battle with that *every day*! I like to be happy. The liquid restriction is the hardest part. I'm always a little thirsty. Plus I like instant gratification, so if I'm thirsty I like to drink! But if I drink a lot, of course, I have a worse dialysis session. When you put on too much liquid, they set the machine to take off more liquid more quickly. Your blood pressure can drop and you can suffer from cramping. This is not pleasant at all; you feel awful. It is best not to do it. I would advise anybody, try your *very best not to drink too much!*"

Do you do anything in your routine that makes dialysis easier?

"First of all, I like to come when the soap operas are on. That makes dialysis go faster for me. Next—and now you are going to laugh at me when I tell you this—I lead a double life. When I leave dialysis I try my best to forget about it. I try very hard not to talk about dialysis or even think about it on the days when I'm not here. Another thing I do is bring along this doggone blanket. It gets cold in here! One more thing that helps with dialysis is building a sense of community at the clinic. I've made an effort. You see these people so many hours every week. Forming relationships with the people here makes it easier to get through this thing. Dialysis seems to be more pleasant too if you know where you are going to be sitting every day and if you get to know your neighbors. That way you have someone to talk to, or borrow money from for lunch or even rely on if something with your treatment is not quite right. If that happens you can tell a neighbor, and they can help get the technician."

What do you do when you aren't at dialysis?

"I'm not one to do a lot of things recreationally. Most activities cost money, and I've never had a lot of that. Basically I go to church.

I'm the church treasurer and as the treasurer I get to interact with a lot of people on the days when I'm not here. I like to go to Reno and play the slot machines! Joe and I, we go out to eat all the time. I spend time with my grandkids. I watch them play basketball or take them to play video games. I try to take part in making sure that they are raised properly."

What are the key success factors to living well on dialysis?

"You *have* to keep a positive attitude. When you don't have a positive attitude it just makes it worse. I don't deal in negatives. The negatives hurt too much. I try to tell myself I'm going to be here four hours, and I thank God every time I walk out that door. I consider it a good day every single time I walk out that door. I think it is best to try to smile and get along with people and will usually try to talk to new people when they come in. Just because you are in a bad situation doesn't mean you can't reach out to people. My grandmother always told me 'it doesn't cost you a nickel to be nice to anybody.' Some people don't do very well. They can't deal with dialysis. You can tell who they are, because they don't say much or converse much. They look into outer space and drag out of here."

What have been the biggest challenges about dialysis?

"Sitting in this chair for so long. I like to be up and doing things. I like to be able to do what I want when I want. In the beginning I didn't expect it to be as demanding as it is. Often it's a hassle, waking up, waiting for the cab, getting here, waiting to be called in. The routine can be awful, the monotony of it, sitting in this chair, dealing with these people. And I'm a person who gets along with everybody!"

Have you been hospitalized since starting dialysis?

"Yes once, when I broke my arm. Your bones get very brittle on dialysis. I slipped on some water and broke my arm in multiple places."

Has your love life been affected by dialysis?

"With *my* husband? It hasn't affected him at all! He's not on Viagra either! Or if he is on Viagra he didn't tell me about it! No, I'll be honest here, I do get more tired, and I don't feel amorous all the time. My husband does get upset about it. I tell him that I'm just tired. Sometimes you are just tired, and your mind is simply set on feeling better. I don't think he is as satisfied as he could be. I have gotten a little more selfish, but have also learned that sometimes I just need to chill out and go with the flow. I really tried to get him to look at our relationship as a brother and sister relationship instead, but for some reason he wouldn't go for that!"

Have you traveled while on dialysis?

"Sure. I've been to Detroit a couple of times. Ohio. Nevada. I dialyze at different places. I wasn't really nervous. The facilities are so similar. I'm just glad to be able to do it. That's the good thing about dialysis; there are clinics all over. In Detroit it looks like there is a dialysis clinic on every corner. I go to Portland once a month to visit my son and grandson. I always go back to the same clinic there. I'm comfortable there. I'm going to Las Vegas in August. Joe and I won a trip! We also take the grandkids down to Monterey once a year and we take them to Big Sur. This year we're going on a fishing trip. We usually go to the coast on the weekends and I make sure I'm back for dialysis on Monday. One thing I've found about traveling that can be difficult is sometimes you have to share a TV; you aren't the regular so you don't get the remote or the power to choose the program. Plus, you have to go whatever hours they'll take you. If I go at five in the morning I have to adapt. The treatment is longer for me without my soap operas to watch."

Any parting words that you think would be helpful for people to know?

"A lot of people in my church know that I'm on dialysis, but I believe they wonder why I'm still walking around. Nobody understands what dialysis is until they sit down in this chair. Recently I read a quote by a little girl with kidney failure who said, 'I wonder why they call it dialysis instead of life-alysis.' I wonder about that too."

Now that the interview has concluded, Susan thanks Donna for her time and asks what Joe is bringing today for lunch. "A ham sandwich," she says then adds, "Sometimes you get tired of sandwiches in here too." She smiles, chuckles, and flips on the overhead television to her favorite soap opera, appropriately titled *One Life to Live*.

Shedding Light on Our Most Common Misperceptions about Dialysis

As Donna's story reflects, most of the world knows very little—or even nothing at all—about renal dialysis and that probably includes or included you once upon a time. The average person on the street might be able to tell you that it is a medical procedure, but chances are that most people know about as much about dialysis as they do about nuclear fusion. What it is exactly, who it affects, and how it is used are rather vague concepts for most of us who've had very little reason to learn about kidney disease.

This relative ignorance really is not a problem, provided you or someone you love doesn't ever actually *need* dialysis. Surprisingly enough, though, according to estimates by the National Kidney Foundation, in 2006 one in nine people in the United States suffer from kidney disease and almost half of these people don't even know it.[1] Contrary to Donna's experience, dialysis has a tendency to sneak up on many people without much or even any warning at all. As another patient reflected, "When I was first diagnosed, I just thought that I had the flu. I was running a fever all the time and feeling tired. I went to the doctor thinking she'd give me some medicine, and I'd be fine. Instead, the doctor figured out that my kidneys were failing and put me on dialysis immediately. I was *really* scared. I didn't know a thing about dialysis. I even told my husband he'd probably have to divorce me, because I was going to be on dialysis. Looking back now, I realize I really didn't have a clue what it meant." Sixteen years later she is still happily married and living on dialysis. Her story is a perfect example of how a general lack of knowledge combined with an unexpected introduction to dialysis can lead us to arrive at mistaken and upsetting conclusions. Family members and patients new to dialysis many times rely on misinformation or pieced-together notions of what they vaguely know or have heard about dialysis. This is completely understandable. But for those who are new to dialysis, this is not particularly helpful and can be frightening.

Amazingly enough, stories of being blindsided by dialysis are not uncommon. But what about the people who have been told in advance that they may have to go on dialysis at some point in the future? Aren't they more informed and less frightened when the rubber finally meets the road? As we saw with Donna, this is not necessarily the case. Denial is a very powerful thing. And for better or worse, many people choose not to learn about dialysis until it is no longer unavoidable and they find themselves hooked up to a machine. That leaves them in the very same predicament as the woman who equated dialysis with divorce: knowing very little and, in many cases, assuming the worst.

Another example of this is our friend Jim, whom we've met through dialysis. Jim is a middle-aged gentleman with a high-school education who went on to become a very successful self-made businessman. He admitted to us that the first time he received dialysis he didn't understand what was happening. He had neither read about dialysis nor been given a thorough introduction to it by the medical professionals he'd met. In fact, as he watched his very lifeblood leaving his body, an overwhelming sense of fear came over him. He imagined it was departing, never to return again. At that very moment he tells us he flat out wanted to die.

Watching his blood being sucked out of his body and not understanding where it was going or what the machine was doing with it, Jim felt lifeless, helpless, lost. He couldn't imagine that a life dependent on a machine was worth living. It sounds quite bleak. But the important take-away message is that Jim had very little information about dialysis. All he had were the sights and sounds of that first treatment. Other than that he was really very much in the dark. The good news is that you don't have to be. The more you know the more you will be able to approach dialysis for what it is: a life-saver, not a life-ender.

Another patient told us that the first doctor who explained dialysis to him described it as "being attached to a machine for the rest of your life." Again this patient thought in literal terms, and for him this was a terrifying statement. The idea of literally lugging around a machine day and night can depress the hell out of even the most optimistic of individuals.

If someone just told us straight up what dialysis is all about, maybe then it wouldn't be so frightening, confusing, or overwhelming. So let's turn the tables on the most common misperceptions and tell it like it is. You might be surprised to hear a realistic depiction of what life on dialysis is really like.

Misperception #1 (The biggest one of them all): Kidney disease is a death sentence.
I'm done. Finished. Finito. Adios. See ya. That's probably what crossed your mind at one point or another when you heard the doctors use the words "End Stage Renal Disease" (ESRD) to describe your irreversible kidney failure. Who can blame you? It's not a huge leap from "end stage" to "the end."

Reality #1: Your life is not over. You are simply beginning a new chapter.
In this age of politically correct terms, it is astonishing that "end stage" is still prevalently being used to describe definitive kidney failure.

In our interviews with many renal health care professionals and patients, we asked if they felt that "end stage" was an accurate term for the
disease. What we often heard back was "Absolutely not!" Most went on
to emphatically say that kidney failure and dialysis are not death sentences. This is really, really important so in case you are skimming this
book we are going to say it again: *Kidney failure and dialysis are not
death sentences!* If you are brand new to dialysis this should be your
mantra for the first six months. You should also remind yourself repeatedly that no one has died and especially not you. In fact, whether
you believe it or not, dialysis is providing you with a new lease on life.
How you use this new lease is in a large part going to be up to you.

The dialysis patients we interviewed prior to writing this book
worked, studied, bore children, raised children, traveled, volunteered,
loved, and lived all the while undergoing hemodialysis three times a
week or peritoneal dialysis daily. When asked what they would tell
patients new to dialysis, several said, "I'd tell them that it is going to
be OK." Or as one patient who'd lived for years via transplant and
dialysis so eloquently put it, "You can be greater than your illness.
You can live with this. It is not the death sentence that it was years
ago. And as technology improves your life can get better."

Now that we've acknowledged that the term End Stage Renal
Disease is a misperception waiting to happen, what to do about
it? Labels and names can have a powerful influence on our self-
perceptions. In fact, we think it's time to do away with "end stage."
Instead, for the purpose of this book and for your mental well-being,
we choose to call it "nonfunctioning kidney disease." We find this to
be a much more appropriate title, because as the patients we met
would tell you, and as their stories throughout this book will show
you, you can live a full and wonderful life without the use of your
kidneys.

True. Your life will change. Significantly. Many patients and medical professionals have likened dialysis to a second job—a very important job that you must take incredibly seriously and always show

up for. This is extremely difficult for many people to digest at first, but with time you will become accustomed to this lifestyle change. For those of you who have children, you could compare this transition to what you experienced in your life before kids versus your life after kids. Just like a new infant who arrives in your home and suddenly becomes a top priority in terms of your time, attention, and care, so now does your dialysis treatment.

Suddenly your life is no longer solely dictated on your terms. Spontaneity takes a back seat to planning, timing, and scheduling. You will need to spend many hours a week devoted to the maintenance of your health. You will likely need to change what you eat and drink. Minor infections and illnesses may have a greater effect on you than on an otherwise healthy individual. You will have good days and not so good days, but the thing to remember is you will have good days. Many of them. In fact, as each year passes, more individuals are able to live longer, fuller lives despite kidney failure. As our friend Jim found out over time, life went on and dialysis wasn't his entire existence. He was even able to continue traveling and having success in his line of work. However, he looks back now on his introduction to dialysis and wishes he had been more informed from the start.

The key to enjoying life even while on dialysis is to focus your attention and energies on the time spent away from dialysis, just as Donna does by leading her so-called double-life. As another example, Daniel spends nine hours weekly on hemodialysis. In addition, he has about four hours of recovery time after each of his dialysis sessions. That equates to a total of twenty-one hours a week spent on dialysis or recovery from dialysis. Here is the bottom line: less than one day out of his week is spent on expending physical or mental energy on dialysis. Daniel takes an out-of-sight, out-of-mind approach. He chooses not to think about dialysis except during those hours. All the other hours, or six days a week, are spent focusing on his family, friends, work, and play. When you put it in those terms, the six days a week made possible by dialysis, as opposed to the zero days that would result without treatment, are a fairly good deal.

Of course, every individual is different and Daniel is just one example of someone living with dialysis. There are individuals who are battling extremely debilitating chronic illnesses or who have significant difficulties with tolerating the permanent accesses for hemodialysis, also known as fistulas or grafts, or who continuously fall ill with infections from peritoneal dialysis. We don't want to minimize the seriousness of their trials. Unlike them, Daniel is comparatively healthy. His veins are able to accommodate a permanent access and he tolerates hemodialysis well. Aside from his lack of kidney function, he is relatively illness free. If luck is on your side and the complications you face are minimal, your experience might not be entirely different from his. Of the patients who do well on dialysis, they will all tell you that keeping busy and having other interests outside of dialysis—friends, family, work, or hobbies—is the key to their success.

And what about the idea that you will be attached to a machine the rest of your life? Well, depending on the form of treatment that you and your doctors select, you will be attached to a machine for a number of hours weekly until a time, should you so choose and be eligible, that you receive a successful transplant. That is the truth. You will need to organize your life in order to be able to access these machines as needed. You won't have the flexibility you once enjoyed to do what you want whenever you want. But with a bit of planning and juggling you will find that much of what you'd like to do can be accommodated. And the truth is you will not be 100% attached to the machine morning, noon, and night, seven days a week, fifty-two weeks a year. In reality it is, as an example, more like nine to twelve hours weekly if you are on hemodialysis or every night while you sleep if you perform a type of peritoneal dialysis. Although not preferable, not something you wished for, or as one patient said, "not something you'd wish upon your worst enemy," this is manageable. Or as another patient told us, "At some point, I realized that the days between treatments I was able to do things that I'd not been able to do before I started dialysis. So I had this every-other-day life and I had my weekends. I think you start from this very narrow picture and as you feel better the lens widens."

Misperception #2: Dialysis is to be feared and is a total downer.

Watching your blood exit and reenter your body through needles and tubes will initially frighten and depress you. Especially in the beginning when you are becoming accustomed to your new routine, it is easier than not to define yourself as a dialysis patient first and a human being second.

Visiting a dialysis clinic is also sobering and frightening at times. You may encounter elderly patients who are senile. You may see individuals who are suffering from a variety of serious illnesses that have resulted in their kidney failure. Some may have amputated limbs and others may have lost their hair. Again, being surrounded by so much illness, it is hard not to feel like an invalid. Why else would you be there if you did not have something seriously wrong with you? And if something is seriously wrong with you, then isn't that now your most self-defining characteristic?

It is not a huge jump from fear to depression. We'd be naive not to acknowledge how easy it is to feel sorry for yourself under the circumstances. In fact, we've been there, as have many of your fellow dialysis patients. You may be anxious about the future and about whether you will live or die. You may be anxious and depressed about how others will perceive you. If you are a sick person, won't everyone treat you like a sick person, someone less than you really are? If going forward, your new role is to be a dialysis patient first and foremost, then what about the person you used to be? You may be upset about your dietary and liquid restrictions. You may also be angry about the fact that you got stuck with this raw deal. Of all people, why you? Why kidney failure?

Reality #2: Dialysis is keeping you alive. You do not need to be defined by your illness.

Just about every individual who goes on dialysis will ponder these questions at one point or another. Of course, there are a few eternal optimists—we've even met a few—who never let dialysis get them down. But if you aren't in that camp you should know that all of these emotions are 100% normal. The key here is not to get stuck in a rut and to dwell on them. Later in the book we will discuss how to conquer these emotions or at the very least mute them. In the meantime, let's present an alternative view.

Just because you are on dialysis doesn't mean you are now simply a dialysis patient waiting around for a miracle cure to jumpstart your life. If you are waiting, you are likely wasting valuable time. It is important to remember that your kidney function is one part of a much bigger whole. Before your kidneys failed you, you probably had many qualities and interests that defined you as a person. Perhaps you loved to cook or to dance, or you were an avid sports fan, a loving parent or grandparent. Now that you use a machine to perform a function that your kidneys used to do, does all or even any of that need to change? For the most part, probably not. Chances are you can still do most of the things that make you who you are. Similarly if you do not obsess about dialysis, talk about it all the time, make it your entire reason for being, those around you won't think about it much either.

We aren't advocating that you don't talk about the changes that you are going through, but it is important to be aware of the line that exists between therapeutically talking and wallowing. Much of what you are experiencing is out of your realm of control, but your attitude and the way you react to these challenges are something you can control. As one dialysis technician told us, "The patients who do well on dialysis bring a positive attitude with them when they walk in the door. Conversely the ones who don't do well and really struggle with dialysis just can't seem to leave the pity-party behind."

Going to dialysis may broaden your horizons and test your ability to be positive in the face of adversity. It may give you a different perspective on life, albeit sometimes a legitimately sad and depressing one. But one thing is certain: dialysis will enable you to keep on living, doing many of the things that you enjoy, and spending time with those you love, for which most dialysis patients eventually are extremely grateful.

Misperception #3: Your only hope for regaining a meaningful life is to receive a kidney transplant.

For most doctors and other medical professionals, as well as for patients, the preferred form of treatment for irreversible kidney failure is a successful kidney transplant. As one doctor said about transplantation, "There is no doubt based on excellent national statistics that the quality of life is improved, the health of the patient is better, and longevity or prognosis for life is extended." But as Donna pointed out, not everyone is a candidate for transplantation and everyone needs to be evaluated as an individual. If you are ineligible or if you are in fact eligible and are then put on a waiting list to receive a new kidney, what does that mean for you in the meantime? Should you put your life on hold?

Reality #3: The more you live now, even without a transplant, the better you will do emotionally.

A discussion of dialysis and transplantation go hand in hand. Dialysis can be life sustaining, as can a successful kidney transplant. Both are the only two viable solutions when dealing with chronic, irreversible kidney failure. Making the decision about whether to pursue a transplant is an important one, and it is something that every dialysis patient should consider and weigh carefully. If you, your family members, and your doctors decide that a transplant will indeed improve your quality and longevity of life, then it is important to remember that it will likely take time for a match to be identified. In the past, transplant patients would hope that an appropriate nonliving donor would eventually be identified. More recently, though, the medical arena is seeing an increasing rise in related and nonrelated living kidney donors, which for certain fortunate individuals may decrease the amount of time spent waiting to locate a match. Waits can range from days to months to years, but the norm for most waits is years. Therefore, even if you are pursuing a transplant and are looking forward to one with great anticipation, a complete understanding of dialysis and how best to live while on dialysis will serve you well until a match is found. If you are always living for the future, you may be missing out on opportunities for joy and satisfaction in the present.

Remember the fairytale tune that starts, "One day my prince will come." Eventually the prince does come. He rescues the princess and finally they live happily ever after. Supposedly she was unhappy—or fully asleep—until he showed up. Does this seem like a waste to you? Snoozing away your life waiting for the prince to show up? Well, the same is true for a successful transplant. Optimists at heart, we hope you will get that much desired and awaited happier ending should you choose to be placed on a transplant list. But in the interim, dialysis is very much keeping you alive. So *now* is the time to be living.

Misperception #4: Your medical care is dictated to you.

Most of us are accustomed to deferring to authority figures. We learn to do this at a young age with our teachers and our parents. If someone is trained to know more than we do, we often assume that knowing more automatically means knowing best.

We also often believe that we have no control over our circumstances. In your case, for whatever reason, your kidneys have failed and that unfortunate event was out of your control. Surely whatever else happens to your health in the future must be equally out of your control.

Reality #4: Not so! You are an active participant in determining and managing your medical care.

Doctors and medical professionals who work with renal patients aren't always perfect. As with any profession, the range of caregivers in renal services can vary from outstanding to poor. And so it is important to remember that when it comes to your health care and your physical well-being, *your number one advocate is you.* As we saw with Donna, she made it her business to learn about the different levels of care that existed at different facilities. When she felt that her facility was less than optimal, she took control and made a change, and as a result she was much happier and more comfortable with life on dialysis.

Bear in mind, most medical professionals are excellent and have only your best interest at heart. However, when you are relying on a machine for survival, the more you know about the machine and your care, the better you will be able to assist and partner with the medical professionals around you. Rather than looking at dialysis as something that is administered to a patient by authority figures, it is best to shift our mind-set to view it as a partnership between patient, technology, and medical professionals.

One dialysis technician mentioned to us that because dialysis affects a large percentage of individuals in the Hispanic community, there are sometimes cultural biases that stand in the way of this mental shift. This particular technician was Hispanic himself. He was very involved in educating his local community about dialysis and nutritional prevention as well as in lobbying for federal funding for food subsidies specific to dialysis patients' needs. In his view, individuals in the Hispanic community who are either new to the United States or are first generation U.S. citizens are so grateful that dialysis is even available that they sometimes don't feel entitled to challenge or raise questions about their quality of care. Whether or not you are a member of this community, you may find yourself feeling this way as well. If so, we recommend that you work to overcome these views. This is after all your life and you are absolutely entitled to speak up on your behalf.

You also have a responsibility to take charge of the daily aspects of your life over which you do have control. The machine can make up for only a small percentage of what would be considered regular kidney function. While you'll never regain a level of function akin to someone with kidneys working at 100% capacity, the remaining percentage of functional improvement is largely dependent on how well you manage your diet and fluids. You can, in other words, do a lot to make your quality of life better. And just as managing your diet and your liquids is in your hands, you also have considerable control over the doctor you see, the clinic you frequent, and the treatment options you choose.

The patients, doctors, technicians, social workers, and dieticians that we interviewed all consistently told us that the more a person learns, asks questions, and actively participates in his or her care, the better the person does both physically and emotionally. You are putting yourself and your life into the hands of others on a daily and weekly basis. As a result, many patients find that the more they understand about the actual machine and the process, the more they are able to relax and to feel less anxious about their treatment. For example, one woman we met said that when she first went on dialysis she wanted to know everything she could about the machine. Having worked as a medical technician herself, she asked to read the technical manual. She read it cover to cover and now understands what any particular beep or ring means. She says knowing this information has put a great number of her fears at ease. This is an extraordinary example and we certainly don't think every dialysis patient needs to do the same. However, we do advocate that, like this patient, you take whatever steps are necessary to make yourself feel more comfortable.

Another dialysis veteran told us he would give these words of advice to someone new to dialysis: "Get as much information as you can. There are a lot of things that will be done for you and to you that are not always explained very well. Make sure that when you are having your initial appointments about dialysis that you have someone there with you who can keep track of everything that is being said. Really get a handle on the labs that they give to you. Understand what they mean. Ask questions and educate yourself as much as you can." Of course, you can't expect to fully control or administer your treatment and at some point you will have to put a certain amount of trust in the professionals and let go. (Or you will be in jeopardy of driving your nurses and technicians batty!) But at the same time, trust your instincts. If you are concerned about something, absolutely feel free to ask questions.

Many other patients echoed this advice and told us they had learned to continuously ask the nurses and technicians questions about what they were doing and why they were doing it, until these patients eventually amassed personal libraries of knowledge sufficiently comforting for them. Some patients mentioned that being educated about their typical dialysis settings and requirements made it easier for them to travel and receive dialysis at other clinics. Why? Because they felt they knew enough to be able to speak up if they sensed that the care or treatment they were receiving didn't mirror the same experience that they were accustomed to at home.

Misperception #5: You can no longer work or study.
Prior to beginning dialysis treatments you may have been feeling worse and worse as your health declined. Depending on the kind of dialysis treatment you choose, you may find that the time needed to tend to your health and recover from your treatments cuts into your regular work or study schedule. Many dialysis patients suffer from serious illnesses that are the cause, rather than the result, of their kidney failure. For them, often their illness or pain can be debilitating

and may prevent them from working. Many elderly individuals, who are well beyond retirement, may suffer from kidney failure. In their case, work or study is not as relevant. The combination of these two groups of individuals can skew the national statistics to appear as if work and study are not an option for many or most renal patients. Again, this can be misleading.

Reality #5: Many dialysis patients do continue to work or study.

When you go to a dialysis clinic and speak with many of the people who fall within the age group of the working population, you will find that a significant number of them manage to work, study, and raise children despite the restrictions that dialysis places on them. And you'll find many patients who cannot work for hire but seek out volunteer opportunities that enable them to grow as human beings, keep their minds active, and help others.

Culinary student, insurance adjustor, pastor, architect, construction worker, retail manager, volunteer, full-time mother, doctor, salesman— these are just some of the professions we encountered when talking with different dialysis patients. Dialysis doesn't mean that you'll have to sit home all day and watch television. One nurse who works with hundreds of dialysis patients told us that of the dialysis patients she encounters, she estimates about one-third work, one-third could be contributing but are not, and the final third truly are unable to do anything. This nurse emphatically said,

> Diagnosis of kidney failure does not indicate disability. For example, if you are young and have polycystic kidney disease, but the rest of your body is in relatively good shape, then why *can't* you work? Work is good for you and for the country. On the other hand, someone who has multiple issues, maybe no legs or chronic infections, and is in and out of the hospital— sometimes in more than out—that person isn't going to work. In those cases disability is justifiable. Sometimes patients give

up too quickly and decide too quickly that they don't want to work. It is important for caregivers to ask their loved ones, "When are you going back to work? When are you going back to school?" If we treat people like invalids they are more inclined to become invalids.

You may, however, need to make some adjustments to your work schedule in an effort to accommodate your treatments. Or you may be in a line of work that you simply find you can no longer do. First, know that you can likely still earn money, and at the very least, you can still do something that enables you to grow or be a contributing member of society and your family. Donna, as a committed volunteer, was a testament to this fact. Scores of dialysis patients derive excellent self-esteem and an abundance of joy from their work. Or as one gentleman reflected on his life on dialysis,

> I wanted to maintain as normal a schedule as I could and I did *not* want to go on disability. I spoke with some people who were enjoying themselves on disability and I thought "how in the world do you do that? That sounds like retirement and I'm too young to retire!" It made a world of difference for me to keep my job. It helped me maintain my sense of worth, kept my income up and preserved a strong sense of identity. Having work that was still vital helped me to know that I was still OK.

Some days you may literally have to drag yourself to where you need to be, but if you can tough those particular days out, overall the emotional benefits of working or volunteering far outweigh the negatives.

Misperception #6: Traveling is out. You are grounded for life.
   In the twenty-first century more and more families find themselves spread around the country and even the world. Where does that leave

you, if you now find yourself on dialysis? How are you going to see your siblings, parents, friends, and children who do not live within driving distance? Will they have to come to you? Or—if you are one of the few lucky ones who have managed to keep all their loved ones close to home—what if you had dreams and aspirations of leisure travel? It will be difficult and frightening to leave the comfort of your dialysis routine at home. Traveling "for fun" doesn't sound so appealing anymore, now that you need dialysis to live. The benefits of travel can't possibly outweigh the hassles of finding a clinic, dealing with travel delays when you are tied to a dialysis schedule, or encountering health complications away from the medical team that you know. Therefore, travel must be limited or curtailed entirely.

Jeffrey had been on dialysis for a little over a year when we met him. He was about to become an empty-nester with his second child going off to college the following year. He told us that one of the hardest things for his spouse was to face the possibility that they would no longer be able to do many of the things they had dreamed of doing after the kids were out of the house. This included the freedom to travel. He acknowledged that he knew it could be done, and in fact, he'd gone to a dialysis clinic in Kansas while visiting his father who coincidentally was also on dialysis. But, he said it was scary for him to go to a new place where they did not know him or his dialysis routine. He took a great deal of comfort in the fact that he was going to the clinic where his father was dialyzing. He knew his father's experience there was a good one. That calmed his fears considerably. Although he commented if it hadn't been for that, he didn't know if he would have ventured away from his regular clinic so soon.

Jeffrey's ambivalence to travel and his wife's disappointment over having to shelve some of their dreams are neither uncommon nor difficult to understand. These are all reasonable fears, but again they are largely a fear of the unknown. The more you know about travel, the less likely you may be to put your dreams on hold.

Reality #6: Put those travel shoes back on! You can still travel to most places in the developed world.

Texas, California, New York, Argentina, Mexico, Jamaica, Israel, England, and aboard a ship in the Atlantic Ocean. These are just a few of the places that Daniel has visited and received dialysis treatments. Did you know there are worldwide cruises that offer dialysis on board? Travel while on dialysis can be done and more important, it can even be enjoyed. There is one critical caveat: Medicare will cover only 80% of the cost of dialysis treatments outside of your home state and Medicaid will cover only in-state dialysis. Neither Medicare nor Medicaid will cover international treatments. Therefore, if you are on Medicare and wish to travel outside the United States or your state, you will either have to pay out-of-pocket for all or a portion of the bill, which can be very costly and for most people is not possible, or you will need to have a secondary insurance program that provides coverage. Again, for many people this is not an option given the associated costs. Depending on your financial situation, you may have to limit your travel to the United States or to your home state. Fortunately we live in a great, gorgeous country with an abundance of wonderful destinations and opportunities for exploration in every state.

If you love to travel or if you have to travel, doing so while on dialysis is not an activity for you to dread or avoid. Plus, the more you make it your business to know your dialysis routine and to manage your care at home, the more empowered you will be to go out on the road. While you may feel your clinic is the only one that will make sure you are well cared for, in reality there are extremely competent dialysis professionals and clinics all over the world. Additionally, there are travel professionals and others who will go the extra mile to help you get your treatments should travel delays occur.

Perhaps you saw coverage during the 2004 Winter Olympics of U.S. Olympic sprinter, Lauryn Williams, whose father traveled to Greece to see her compete. Despite his dialysis requirements David Williams wasn't going to miss attending his daughter's competition.[2] The television crews documented him walking into a dialysis clinic in Athens and then cut back to him in the stands cheering her on. Now you might be thinking, "Well, if I had a daughter competing in the Olympics too, then *sure* I'd travel for *that*. But it isn't happening, so I'm staying put." The point is, even if you just want to visit Florida in the winter for no other reason than to get out of the cold, or you want to visit your niece who is celebrating her third birthday, those are reasons enough. You don't live to dialyze. You dialyze to live. If you pass up opportunities to do the things you have dreamed of, then dialysis isn't serving its intended purpose.

Certainly there are some remote or unsafe places that you won't be able to visit like the boundary waters between the United States and Canada or Antarctica, but we assure you there are plenty of fabulous destinations left for you to go to easily. Sometimes we think if we stick with the routine that is most familiar we will be safe and in control. The truth is, if you are on dialysis or not, staying at home and in your routine does not ensure that you will be safe or healthy. Getting out and seeing the world or those you love, should you have the desire, does ensure that you are making the most of the present. Later in the book we will provide tips and tricks on how to minimize your fears of the unknown when traveling and to create contingency plans should anything go awry while you are on the road.

We hope that much of what you've read so far resonates with your experiences or at the very least has provided you with helpful insight into many of the generalizations surrounding dialysis—the good, the bad, and the ugly—but we don't intend to stop here. Several other patients and medical professionals have shared their stories with us. Each of their tales provides excellent ideas and suggestions for living well on dialysis despite the very real challenges and the sometimes not so real ideas surrounding this medical treatment. Now that you have read both the loftiest and the most detrimental misconceptions that exist, we hope you will be inclined to ignore them as much as possible. But if you do find yourself listening to them, try to remember the sage words of advice shared by many dialysis veterans, "It is going to be OK."

Two

A Visit to the Suds Factory

Demystifying the Machines and Tubes

FOR MOST PEOPLE, going to a hemodialysis center for the first time is a bit frightening and overwhelming. This is true for both patients and the family members who may be accompanying them. The tubes, machines, blood, and needles can be daunting to a first-timer. In fact, it can be daunting for a good while. So we wondered how we could take away some of the fear factor.

We once knew a young boy who was scheduled for a tonsillectomy. Before the big day arrived his father took him to an orientation at the children's hospital. The boy was able to put on gowns and gloves, to taste the different flavors used for the anesthesia, and to see the tricycle that he would ride into the operating room. The goals of this show-and-tell were to mentally prepare the boy and to ease his fears of the unknown. Just because adults are older doesn't mean they are any less frightened when it comes to undergoing medical procedures. Shouldn't people young and old alike receive an orientation of what takes place in the dialysis clinic?

Many centers do provide educational guidance and tours to patients before they first start dialysis. Ideally, all patients new to dialysis will have at least visited a center before they dialyze for the first time so that they have a chance to absorb their surroundings and ask questions about the procedure ahead of time. Realistically, however, many patients never tour a clinic or attend a class before their initial treatment. Or, even if they do, they may be too sick, overwhelmed, or inhibited to inquire at length about the sights and sounds around them. So we thought we'd provide a step-by-step account of what it is like to go through a hemodialysis session at a center—or as we humorously like to call it, the suds factory, because it is, after all, where a dialysis patient goes to get "clean."

In-center hemodialysis is far and away the most common type of dialysis at present. To receive this type of dialysis a patient needs to travel to a center, arriving at an appointed time assigned by the center's staff. Centers are located in towns and cities all over the United States and the world. Typically, visits are scheduled three times weekly on Mondays, Wednesdays, and Fridays or on Tuesdays, Thursdays, and Saturdays. Most people will dialyze for three to four hours each session, although some may dialyze longer. Even if you plan to pursue peritoneal dialysis or a transplant (see Chapters 3 and 4 for explanations and discussions of these alternative treatments), it is highly likely that you will spend a period of time hemodialyzing in a center, so our tour is recommended for all kidney patients and family members who wish to understand more about what takes place there and why.

On this verbal tour we'll try to describe and explain the before, during, and after of a visit to the suds factory. We'll cover a variety of topics from what to bring with you, to why you step on the scale, to how the machine works as an artificial kidney, to what happens when the technicians remove the needles at the end of the session. And at the end of the tour, we will share the perspective of a key figure in every clinic, a dialysis nurse.

Before Dialysis

Understanding the Role of Kidneys and What Happens When They Fail

Before you walk into a hemodialysis center you must be contending with one inescapable truth: your kidneys are no longer functioning properly, and as a result your health is deteriorating. Therefore, our first stop on this tour is to understand just what happens to you as your kidneys tucker out.

Typically healthy kidneys perform four important jobs:

1. Filter and remove excess fluid from the blood.

2. Filter and remove toxic impurities or waste products from the blood.

3. Produce hormones that help control blood pressure, make red blood cells, and promote absorption of calcium from the intestines to strengthen bones.

4. Balance mineral and chemical levels in your body such as sodium, potassium, calcium, and phosphorus.

As healthy kidneys filter out excess fluid and waste products from the blood, they create urine. These harmful excess fluids and toxins are then flushed from your body every time you urinate. But as your kidney function decreases, so does your output of urine. Your body begins stockpiling unhealthy amounts of poisons and liquid. One of the major poisons is urea. The condition associated with a buildup of urea is called uremia. Poor appetite, nausea, vomiting, itching, fatigue, and confusion are some of the most common symptoms of uremia.

In addition to this abundance of urea, you are carrying around extra liquid, which is adding stress to your heart. At first, this excess liquid is being stored in your bloodstream. When your bloodstream fills to capacity, liquid begins moving into your cells and tissues, which can cause edema, uncomfortable bloating, and swelling throughout your body. Eventually excess liquid can even build up in your lungs, creating respiratory distress. At the same time, your production of erythropoietin, the hormone healthy kidneys create to signal the production of red blood cells, is diminishing and you are becoming increasingly anemic. Being anemic can be likened to trying to drive a car without any gas; you lack the energy reserves necessary to run.

No wonder most people feel like they've been run over by a Mack truck prior to beginning treatment. Starting to panic? Don't. Instead, appreciate the fact that now there is a scientific man-made filtration system—dialysis. Undergoing dialysis, and receiving modern-day medications such as a pharmaceutical replacement for erythropoietin, can significantly improve your health.

Unfortunately, dialysis is not as effective as having a healthy kidney, but it can get you part of the way there. As one doctor remarked, "Dialysis can only remove approximately 10% to 15% of the toxins that normal kidneys can. Patients' ability to adapt their diet, manage their liquid intake and take their medicines plays on the ability of the dialysis technology to give them a reasonably comfortable and successful life." The dialysis technology cannot do it all. In order to live well while on dialysis, you will need to do some of the work.

As your kidney health declines prior to beginning dialysis, your nephrologist can use a mathematical formula based on a number of factors, such as your age, gender, ethnicity, and blood level of creatinine (waste product of muscle metabolism, a chemical measure of kidney health) to determine your glomerular filtration rate (GFR), which is essentially a measurement of the health of the kidneys. There are five stages of kidney disease as defined by GFR:

Stage 1: kidney damage with normal GFR of 90 or above.

Stage 2: kidney damage with mild decrease in GFR at 60–89—as an example, those who are hypertensive or diabetic may be in this stage for years and years.

Stage 3: moderate decrease in GFR 30–59.

Stage 4: severe reduction in GFR 15–29—at this stage you may live without dialysis but your health may bottom out from under you very quickly. Despite this, some people live comfortably at this stage for a very long time.

Stage 5: kidney failure GFR rate of less than 15—a person needs to be on dialysis or receive a transplant to live.

The Goals of Hemodialysis

In preparation for your visit to the hemodialysis center, you should have a basic understanding of the goals of this medical procedure. They are twofold: first to filter and remove the toxic impurities that have built up in your blood and second to filter and remove the excess liquid that has built up in your body. To achieve these goals, your blood will quite literally be removed from your body, cleansed by a machine, also referred to as a dialyzer or an artificial kidney, and then returned back to your body. Only about one cup of blood will be outside of your body at any time during this process, and you will not experience any feeling or sensation of blood exiting or reentering your body.

An Introduction to Your Lifeline

In order to receive hemodialysis, you will need to have an access, also sometimes referred to as a "lifeline," built to deliver enough blood to the dialyzer for cleansing. Your access is the site where your blood will exit and reenter your body. There are two categories of accesses: "permanent" and "temporary." First, let's outline the major differences between these two categories:

1. Most important, permanent accesses allow for more efficient dialysis by providing a greater blood flow than do temporary accesses. This means that often patients will feel substantially better if they are dialyzed with the use of a permanent access.

2. Permanent accesses also have decreased risks of infection and last much longer than temporary accesses.

3. Permanent accesses require minor outpatient surgery and ample time to fully become established and heal before they can be put to use. Temporary accesses can be used immediately.

4. Permanent accesses are typically constructed in a patient's forearm but can be created in the upper arm or leg as well. Temporary accesses are placed in the neck or groin.

For long-term treatment, permanent accesses are the preferred option. Ideally, patients will be followed by a physician throughout the course of their renal decline and will have a permanent access created several months in advance of when they will actually need to begin hemodialysis. Of course, many people are not followed carefully, or their final renal decline happens faster than anticipated, or their illness isn't discovered until they need dialysis immediately. In those cases a temporary access is the next best option. Now that you understand the major differences between a permanent and a temporary access, let's explore the specific types of accesses within each category.

Permanent Hemodialysis Accesses

There are two main types of permanent accesses—arteriovenous (AV) fistulas and grafts. To understand the differences between the two, we must first understand the primary difference between an artery and a vein. An artery is a blood vessel that carries blood away from the heart. A vein is a blood vessel that carries blood toward the heart. Imagine two parallel highways transporting your blood in different directions. The most efficient way to improve the rate of blood flow in and out of your body during dialysis is to connect these two highways. How these highways beneath your skin are connected is the primary difference between a fistula and a graft.

Imagine a vascular surgeon pulls the parallel highways together so that they somewhat resemble an X. The vein and artery are now connected directly at the center of the X. This is essentially what an AV fistula looks like beneath your skin. Now imagine a vascular surgeon attaches an artery indirectly to a vein by using a small plastic tube. In this case, the actual connection between the two highways resembles more of a U shape with the highways running lengthwise up and down each side of the U. This is essentially what an AV graft looks like beneath your skin. In the end, a fistula or graft may or may not exactly resemble the X and U configurations above, but we use these examples to help you visualize the constructive differences between the two.

Other important differences between fistulas and grafts are these:

1. Usually it takes a few months for the fistula to develop before it can be put to use, whereas a graft is most often ready in a few weeks.

2. On average, fistulas have lower rates of infection and clotting, last longer, and provide better overall performance than grafts.

In general, fistulas are considered to be the best type of permanent vascular access. However, some patients have medical conditions that prevent the use of a fistula. For example, a patient's veins may be too delicate to be connected directly to an artery. In this case and others where a fistula isn't an option, a graft is the next best choice.

A vascular surgeon will decide which type of permanent "lifeline" you are best suited for. The surgeon will perform an outpatient procedure to create your access with the use of a local anesthetic or, as is more common, with intravenous sedation or general anesthesia. You will likely experience some pain and swelling for several days or weeks after undergoing the procedure. In time, your lifeline will be ready for use, and in the interim if you need to be dialyzed a temporary access will be used.

Temporary Hemodialysis Accesses

Temporary accesses are often used when a patient is waiting for a permanent access to heal, when a patient's veins or arteries cannot accommodate a permanent access, or when a patient's permanent access has failed. Even though they are called temporary they remain in place and are not removed until the permanent access is ready for use. A catheter, a flexible hollow tube, is inserted into a vein in the neck or groin. In the neck the catheter may jut out directly or a catheter may exit through the chest via a subcutaneous (under the skin) tunnel that serves to prevent infection. Catheters in the neck or groin must be kept clean and dry at all times, which renders swimming or bathing off limits. Until a permanent access is in place, a patient will need to use a special protective device in order to shower. Last, catheters are then connected to the dialyzer without the use of needles.

Having your permanent access built or your temporary access inserted is a critical step in the "before" part of our tour. Once this has been accomplished you may want to begin thinking about what you would like to bring with you to your dialysis sessions.

Packing a Bag for Dialysis: What to Bring

To assist you in packing a small bag or backpack we've broken our recommendations into four categories: how to stay occupied, comfortable, satisfied, and relaxed.

How to Stay Occupied

Some people like to read, watch TV, do crossword puzzles, listen to music, sleep, work, talk on their cellular phones, even play movies or games on their laptop computers while dialyzing. Think about how you might like to best spend your time. If you think you'd enjoy catching up on some back issues of magazines you've been meaning to read, then by all means pack them up. Or if you find music relaxes you, then perhaps you could bring a CD or MP3 player and headphones with you. These are but a few examples. The point is that planning ahead can make the time go faster.

How to Stay Comfortable

You are going to be sitting for three to four hours so be sure to wear comfortable clothes. Sometimes at the end of a session when you are being taken off the machine, it is not uncommon to get some blood on your clothing. Therefore, we recommend you wear items that are easily washable. Often people will feel cold during a session so feel free to bring a cozy blanket with you. And if you want to try to sleep while you dialyze, you might want to bring a soft pillow for your head.

How to Stay Satisfied

Many times, people are "squeezing" dialysis into a busy schedule, and as a result they might not make it to breakfast or lunch. For this reason and others (for example, diabetics may *have* to eat) many centers allow patients to bring food. Check with your particular center regarding their policy on food, and if they give you the go-ahead, then pack a healthy snack or meal.

How to Stay Relaxed

Last, if you are feeling a little nervous or scared, bring a family member or a friend to keep you company the first few times. Again, you'll need to check with your center regarding their policy toward guests, but most centers will allow guests for different durations of time. If you can't bring one of your nearest and dearest with you, then perhaps bring the next best thing: a few photos of your parents, partner, kids, or grandkids to keep you company, give you comfort, and remind you just why you are sitting in that chair.

A Final Check

Before heading out to dialysis, Daniel always checks the status of his graft. He does this by feeling for a thrill, a vibration, which indicates a pulse. A missing pulse is a sign that the access is not operating correctly. Twice Daniel has arrived at the center and there was no pulse. On those occasions he had to return home without dialyzing and immediately contact his doctor to determine what was wrong and how it could be resolved. Both times Daniel's graft had clotted, meaning that the plastic tube had become clogged with coagulated blood. By performing a fairly simple outpatient procedure, the radiologist unclogged his graft with a medical device just as a plumber would unclog a pipe. Between dialysis sessions, Daniel also checks his access for any sign of infection. If he were to notice any redness, irritation, or tenderness, he would contact his doctor immediately.

The Journey

Health and weather permitting, Daniel prefers to drive himself to the dialysis center. He finds driving himself to be good for his self-esteem and sense of autonomy. Margie also likes when he is able to drive himself, but for different reasons. It makes her role as caretaker less taxing. Over the years, she has adapted to her role well, but she too likes her independence and enjoys when she does not have to shuttle him three days a week. Similar to Daniel, many patients will drive themselves. But the ability to drive does not need to make or break your sense of independence. In fact, we asked one patient how she would manage if she couldn't drive. She just shrugged and said, "Well, if I couldn't drive, I'd take the bus. The bus will take you anywhere you want to go." Many dialysis patients regularly receive rides from family or will take cabs, public transportation, or transportation organized by social services. Determining a reliable and dependable mode of transportation is a critical part of the planning process. The key is to find and arrange for a method of transportation that will consistently get you to the clinic on time. Once this has been accomplished you will be ready to leave home and head to the clinic.

During Dialysis

Waiting

Arriving at the clinic, you will check in at the waiting room. There may be coffee or a place to hang your coat. There will likely be helpful pamphlets, recipes, or other literature available for patients. Some clinics will allow you to simply pass through the waiting room, go directly into the unit, and sit down in your spot. Others will ask you to stay in the waiting room until a technician comes to get you. Many patients do not like having to wait to dialyze. They'd prefer to get started right away. Waiting just adds extra time to the whole process when they'd already rather be somewhere else. On the other hand, waiting rooms also build community. They become places to meet other patients, spouses, and children, learn about their lives, and catch up on how their days are going. Having this sense of community can make time pass more quickly, boost one's spirits, and make the entire experience much more endurable.

Alternatively, one patient told us that he always found himself waiting with a group of individuals who constantly tried to outdo one another with their woes and problems. In time, he found their negativity to be infectious. Finding himself sinking deeper into depression, he decided to switch to a clinic where he could walk straight into the unit and build his nest at his chair without any wait. The point of this story is that there are healthy, positive communities and there are unhealthy, negative communities. If you ever notice yourself being sucked into playing the "who is most miserable" game, perhaps put a bit of distance between yourself and the other contenders. This is one competition that you would be better off not trying to win.

Inside the Unit

As you enter the unit, you may see as few as five chairs or as many as fifty-five. Some clinics may have rows of chairs facing each other. Others may have chairs lining the walls of the room. A chair typically resembles a big Lazy-Boy recliner.

While different centers may have different set-ups, we'll describe what we frequently see at Daniel's clinic. Intravenous (IV) stands are alongside each of the chairs, as are dialysis machines with monitors on top. The technicians and nurses who are working and walking about are usually dressed like nurses in a hospital. At first glance, patients are sleeping, reading, eating, watching TV, and talking on their cell phones. Before he sits down, Daniel's chair will be wiped down with bleach and disinfectant. These cleaning agents create a particular smell, which in time you will notice is common to most centers. Cleanliness in the clinic is important to guard against infection. As patients arrive inside the unit, they are also advised to thoroughly wash their hands.

Weigh In: Determining How Much Water to Take Off

Typically, when you enter the unit, your first order of business will be to weigh in and have your blood pressure checked. This weight is called your "wet" weight or how much you weigh with all the additional fluid you've stockpiled. Like most dialysis patients, you do not urinate to any significant degree. Excess fluid is first stored in your bloodstream. When your bloodstream fills to capacity, then the fluid backs up into the cells and tissues in your body and your blood pressure rises above normal. One of the goals of your dialysis session will be to get you down to your "dry" weight at which your blood pressure is normal; it is the weight you should have without all this additional fluid. To achieve your dry weight, the dialyzer will pull off excess liquid from your bloodstream. As this liquid departs, additional liquid that has seeped into your tissues will now have room to move into your bloodstream. After it enters the bloodstream, it too is then pulled off by the dialyzer.

If you have been amassing fluid over a long time, you might not be able to get down to your dry weight in just one session. It may take several sessions to remove all this additional fluid. But let's say after several initial sessions you arrive at this weight, and for the sake of explanation let's call this your "very first dry weight." This would be the very first time you have been at your proper, normal weight since your kidneys failed. Because the role that your weight plays in dialysis is both a very important and very complex topic that is rarely explained well, let's look at it in some depth here and describe this role in steps.

Step One: Once your very first dry weight is reached, ideally you would maintain this weight forever, never gaining or losing any fat or muscle weight. This is completely unrealistic, but let's say for now that it's possible. We'll call this fat or muscle weight "real kilograms." In medicine, weight is typically measured in kilograms, not pounds, but to give you a frame of reference one kilogram is about 2.2 pounds. Now let's imagine a fantasy world, where the *only* fluctuations in your weight would be from the kilograms you gain from retaining liquid. We'll call these kinds of kilograms "liquid kilograms."

Step Two: Now let's imagine that you live in this fantasy world where you never gain or lose real weight and your very first dry weight, after dialyzing on Monday, is 70 kilograms (abbreviated kgs.). On Wednesday, when you arrive for your next session you step on the scale so the technician can determine your wet weight. You weigh 72.5 kgs. This is your wet weight. The difference between your dry and wet weight is 2.5 kgs. We know, because we live in the world of fantasy, that all 2.5 of these kilograms are liquid. So, the dialysis machine will be set to remove 2.5 kgs. of liquid over the course of your dialysis session. When the 2.5 kgs. have been removed, your technician will know that you are back to your correct dry weight.

Step Three: But here is the catch: you live in the real world where you do gain and lose real kilograms. Now let's imagine that between dialysis sessions you suffer from a lack of appetite and inadvertently lose one real kilogram between Monday and Wednesday. Now your dry weight is really 69 kgs., but you recall Monday's scale that read 70 kgs. On Wednesday, you step on the scale and it reads 72.5 kgs. In reality you've gained 3.5 liquid kilograms. But it appears that you've gained only 2.5 liquid kilograms. After the dialyzer removes the 2.5 kilograms of liquid, how will you and your medical team know that you are actually carrying around one additional kilogram in liquid weight and that your dry weight is now 69 kgs., not 70 kgs.? You'll know because your blood pressure after dialysis will be higher than usual and you may be short of breath. Not enough fluid has been removed. If your blood pressure is still substantially above your normal rate at the end of a session, then you are very likely still retaining too much fluid. The physician may decide to lengthen the session or have more liquid removed at the next session.

Step Four: Now let's envision an alternative real-world scenario. On Tuesday, while celebrating your birthday, you eat too much food, including cake. In this example, without your knowledge or any way to measure it, you gain one real kilogram between Monday and Wednesday. Now your dry weight is really 71 kgs., but you recall the scale read 70 kgs. On Wednesday, when you arrive at the dialysis clinic, you step on the scale and it reads 72.5 kgs. In reality you've gained 1.5 liquid kilograms and one real kilogram, but it appears you've gained 2.5 liquid kilograms. In this case, the dialysis machine will be set to take off too much liquid. What will happen? You may feel light-headed or nauseous and your blood pressure is likely to drop during and after dialysis.

These two examples highlight the fact that determining your correct dry weight is not an exact science. Weighing in does provide

the best estimate of how much liquid to remove, but it is just that—
an estimate. You and your medical team will use a number of indicators both during and after the session to help determine how much
liquid needs to be removed.

How the Machine Works: Determining How Quickly to Remove the Liquid

The technician has an idea of how much fluid to remove. Now how
does he or she know how fast to remove it? In each of the examples
above the technician will set the machine to remove 2.5 kilograms
over the course of the session. But how long will the session be? If 2.5
kilograms is removed over three hours, the rate of removal will be
faster than if it is removed over four hours. In actuality the length of
the session will be prescribed by your physician, but the rate of fluid
removal may vary based on your physical reaction to dialysis. The
rate that fluid moves from the bloodstream into the dialyzer is called
the ultrafiltration rate (UFR). At the same time, fluid moves from
your tissues into the bloodstream. The removal process itself involves
two steps.

Step One: Your blood has several components, two of which are
red blood cells and plasma that together make up your total blood
volume. The plasma contains the excess fluid and toxins that the dialyzer, serving as a sieve, sifts out. Because the red blood cells are
too big to fit through the holes of the sieve, they are left in the
bloodstream.

Step Two: As the dialyzer removes these toxins and fluid from the
plasma, your overall blood volume drops. At the same time, your
blood volume rises as more fluid moves from your tissues and cells
into your bloodstream. You will have an optimal session if your
blood volume does not go too low or too high.

Now that we've introduced you to the scale and to how the machine works, it is time to "go on."

"Going On": Getting Hooked Up to the Dialyzer

After your wet weight is logged, the technician will take your blood pressure. At this point, your blood pressure should be higher than normal because you have additional fluid in your body. Blood pressure and body fluid are usually directly related. This is one reason that people with high blood pressure are told to cut down on salt. Salt causes us to retain fluid, and fluid retention increases blood pressure. Next, the technician cleans your access with alcohol and iodine. At this point, if you have a catheter, the technician connects the catheter, without the use of any needles, directly to the tubes into which your blood will flow. Or, if you have a permanent access, the technician then inserts a very large needle into one side of the permanent access—and by large, we mean quite large. As one patient said to us, "I wish someone had told me that they used sixteen gauge, and I mean *big*, needles. That was a shocker. I would have liked to have known that. I don't know if it would have made me any more comfortable, but it might not have been such a shock."

This needle is attached to plastic tubing that is about twelve inches long. The tube is marked red, which indicates it is the arterial line or the line that removes the "dirty" blood. A second large needle is used to insert another twelve-inch tube into the other side of the access. This tube is marked blue, which indicates it is the venous line or the line that returns the "clean" blood to the body. Your technician may ask which side of your access is red and which is blue. Your doctor will have shown you this in advance. Attached to each of these twelve-inch tubes are two very long, thin clear tubes that connect to the dialysis filter. The filter is a thick, hollow-looking tube that resembles the shaft of a flashlight. It sits alongside the machine in plain view. The dialysis filter is where all the action takes place—that is, where your excess fluid and impurities will be removed from your blood.

Now comes the stick. The needles can be placed at several different points running about three inches along the length of the access.

You should remind the technician to rotate the cannulation site (the site where the needle is inserted to draw off fluids) each time to ensure that you are not stuck in the same place each time. This will allow the site time to recover after a session before it is eventually reused.

There are topical anesthetics, such as Lidocaine or Emla, that can be used to numb the access. Whether these creams are prescription or over-the-counter varies by state. Applied at least a half hour before treatment, these ointments prevent you from feeling any pain from the needles. In addition, you might want to employ breathing or visualization techniques to relax. Sometimes you may get stuck multiple times before the technician is able to successfully connect (not fun). Other times they may connect on the first try (whew!). Once inserted, the needles are taped down. One patient told us that because he had a lot of arm hair, his arm always hurt when the tape was pulled off at the end of a session. He recommended to those in a similar predicament that they carefully shave the hair around the access site so that the untaping will be less painful.

"Being On": What Happens While You Dialyze

Once your access is attached to the dialyzer, the process of cleaning your blood begins immediately. The plastic tubing as it nears the machine jumps constantly. This jump results from the pump on the machine that is continuously circulating your blood. During the dialysis process you will likely hear many beeps coming from the monitors on the machines throughout the room. Your machine will be constantly monitoring several pieces of vital information, including but not limited to your pulse, blood pressure, the amount of water that has been removed, the rate of removal of water, the blood flow rate, and the treatment time. Throughout the session your blood volume may fluctuate.

What happens if your blood volume drops too low? You can "crash" or feel sick. Remember that body liquid and blood pressure are directly related. A drop in blood volume beyond a certain threshold (a tolerance level that is unique to every individual) can lead to a significant drop in blood pressure, followed by cramping, dizziness, lightheadedness, or nausea. If you suffer from any of these symptoms, a technician may lower your UFR or temporarily or permanently stop removing liquid for the remainder of your session. He or she may also inject saline solution directly into your venous line, which will immediately increase your blood volume. This, in turn, will improve your blood pressure. The nurse or technician may adjust your chair so that you are in a reclining position with your head lowered and your feet up. Over time, through trial and error, you and the technicians will learn just how much liquid can be removed and at what rate before you crash.

But what if your blood volume levels are too high while you are dialyzing? That means that the fluid is being removed too slowly. In this instance, the technician may increase the UFR so that fluid will be removed more quickly.

Every individual reacts differently to dialysis and can react differently on any given day. Taking off too much liquid too quickly can make you feel bad. That's why consuming too much liquid between sessions often makes for a more miserable session. Taking off just the right amount at just the right speed should make for an easier session. However, pinpointing the correct amounts and rates of removal is challenging, especially when real and liquid weight gain can fluctuate constantly. Plus, determining a patient's threshold is essentially a "live and learn" process, which is another reason that dialysis can be particularly rough on a patient in the first few months of treatment.

Occasionally patients faint from excessively low blood pressure, causing a medical emergency when the paramedics will be called. The din of the clinic disappears. Everyone is silent. Fortunately, such emergencies are rare. In the seven years that Daniel has been dialyzing, for example, he has witnessed them only a few times. Most of the time, though, it's just business as usual, and a good dialysis session is one that is very uneventful and quite boring. You sit, listen to beeps, and pass the time as pleasantly as you can until your session is over. And like Daniel, you try not to think of these emergencies happening to you.

"Coming Off": Being Unhooked from the Machine

Time passes one way or another. The machine's screen shows how many minutes of treatment remain. Once it is time to "come off" the machine, all of the blood in the dialyzer is returned to your body. The technician puts on gloves and, depending on unit policy, may hand you a glove so that you can assist with the process of stopping the blood flow. The technician begins to pull off the strips of tape that are holding the needles in place, removes the long tubes from the shorter ones, sterilizes the site with an iodine swab, and then pulls the two needles out of the skin. Occasionally there may be an overflow of blood when the needles are removed. The technician places gauze pads over the spots where the needles were and instructs you to press down on the gauze for about ten minutes. The pressure will help the blood to clot.

Sometimes it may take longer for the blood to clot. If you are not strong enough to apply adequate pressure, a plastic cuff can be used to stem the blood flow. You will not be able to leave until the bleeding has stopped. While you continue to press down on your access, the technician cleans out the machine. The long tubes are thrown away. In many clinics the plastic dialyzer is also discarded, while in some the dialyzer may undergo "reuse" in the same patient after cleansing and sterilization (in which case, at the next session, the technician will first show the patient that the filter is entirely clean and clear, without any cleaning residue left inside, before attaching it to the machine). Eventually, after you apply pressure to your access, your blood clots. The technician places tape over a fresh piece of gauze over your access, and for the last time, records your sitting and standing blood pressure and weight. Now it is time to leave.

After Dialysis

How You Will Feel

Different people respond in different ways to dialysis. Some feel absolutely fine after they finish. They get up out of the chair and go on with their day or evening as though they had never been to the clinic. Other people may have a more adverse reaction. They may feel tired or weak. They may suffer from diarrhea, cramping, vomiting, or a general funk for different periods of time after a session.

Daniel experiences something in between. Typically he has plenty of energy to drive himself home. He is always hungry and looks forward to the meal that Marjorie prepares for him. But after dinner he begins to, as he says, "sink." At this point he feels very tired and devoid of energy. He is really not fit to do anything other than watch ESPN or the SCI-FI channel and go to bed. But, when he awakes in the morning he feels great until about nine or ten A.M. when at some point he will experience a shorter slump. For approximately half an hour he will feel very tired, very much like he felt the night before. Then it will pass. This is his typical recovery routine after every session.

It is important, once you determine your typical reaction, to find a schedule that best accommodates your side effects. For instance, if you find that you are useless after dialysis, you may want to try to avoid morning sessions right before you go to work or school and instead schedule afternoon or early evening sessions so that you can go home and sleep. This may not always be possible, but with some advanced planning, your clinic may be able to work with you.

Abnormal Occurrences

On a few occasions Daniel has experienced atypical aftereffects. Once he was acting confused and disoriented (signs of uremia). Another time he suffered from diarrhea, felt very weak, and had trouble sleeping. Because these after effects were abnormal for him, he contacted his doctor and in each case he either returned for more dialysis, altered his diet, or had a longer session the next time. Another atypical occurrence, which he and others at his clinic have experienced, is bleeding from the access site after leaving the unit. This can be both messy and frightening. Sometimes you will have gotten no farther than the parking lot before the bleeding resumes. If you haven't gone far you will need to turn around and head back into the unit for additional assistance. However, if this happens at home you will need to try to stop the bleeding on your own. If you cannot, then you should call your doctor or visit an emergency room.

Life Marches On

Daniel has noticed over the years that the patients who put on too much fluid between sessions typically endure longer and more physically taxing dialysis sessions. They often have more difficulty with side effects after the sessions as well. He is grateful to experience relatively minor aftershocks. The day after he returns home from dialysis he will remove the tape that is covering the gauze on his access. That day he, like thousands of other dialysis patients, may work, exercise, partake in a hobby, talk to his children, enjoy time with his wife. Life marches on. The dialysis session is a thing of the past. This is the after. Maybe not happily ever—but certainly happily enough.

Before we put the suds factory entirely behind us, we'd like to share some parting thoughts and words of wisdom from an important and central figure in every clinic: a nurse. Daniel met this particular nurse, Madeline, at a clinic where he dialyzed while on vacation. The clinic serves over 200 patients and is one of the largest in the United States. Madeline first began working with dialysis patients twenty years earlier while stationed in the intensive care unit (ICU) of a hospital. Eventually she left the ICU to work for a nephrologist's practice where she did rounds in a dialysis clinic. In time, she moved to her current clinic where she started out managing technicians and administering care for patients, then began to oversee new-patient and staff education, and ultimately became the clinic's director. When Daniel and she initially met, she was still in charge of education. Upon hearing of Daniel's book project, Madeline expressed a warm willingness to share much of what she had learned and observed about patients, patient education, and living well on dialysis. She graciously agreed to be interviewed by Susan. Because the two women lived in separate cities, they decided to conduct the interview by phone.

Madeline's Story, a Dialysis Nurse and Educator's Perspective

Susan begins by asking Madeline about her role as the clinic's educator and what that means. Madeline explains that she is responsible for training all the new employees at the clinic, which requires a varying level of instruction depending on the individual. Aside from ensuring that state-mandated standards and continuing education needs for professionals are met, Madeline is also in charge of patient education, which she emphasizes, "is critical for most patients when they first start dialysis."

Madeline explains that for most people, beginning dialysis is the worst thing that has happened to them in their life. At first, people are usually in shock and disbelief and will test their boundaries. They refuse to believe that they can't drink more than a certain amount or that they can't eat whatever they like. Many are for the first time realizing and coming to terms with the idea that they won't live forever. Madeline tells Susan that for many patients, having an educator who can answer questions and provide guidance can ease one's transition to life on dialysis.

Do most people receive education before they begin dialysis?

"Most people do not receive any education before their kidneys fail. Often the kidney failure isn't caught in time, or if it is, the patients still aren't *really* educated. Many of the symptoms of kidney disease aren't things that you would think are related to your kidneys. For example, my brother has had high blood pressure for twenty years, but he didn't take his medications because he didn't feel bad. Over time the unmanaged high blood pressure has taken its toll, and now his kidneys are failing."

In your opinion, what are the key factors or characteristics of patients who do well on dialysis?

"The patients who do well are very active in their care. They don't do well by accident. They are following their diet. They are attending all their treatments. They are not cutting their dialysis time short. They are not bending the rules, or if they are, they aren't doing it frequently. They don't fight with it anymore. I'm not saying that they don't get down or wish that they didn't have to go to that 'damn place,' but they get up in the morning and get out there."

What advice do you give to patients who are new to dialysis?

"When I meet new dialysis patients sometimes they have never been dialyzed or sometimes they have already been dialyzed a few times in the hospital. The first thing that I want them to know is how much power they have. If they choose not to follow their doctor's prescription, that's their own business. But if they don't do it, I want them to know what the consequences will be. I want them to be making an informed decision. You have to be able to shoot straight with the patients; let them know these are their choices and these are the consequences."

Do you ever have patients who don't quite grasp that they must come to dialysis religiously?

"I had one patient who came to dialysis once a week for three weeks. He was carrying around seventy-five pounds of liquid. His legs were so big he could not bend them. A lot of new patients tell me, 'I'm too sick to come to dialysis.' I explain to them that is exactly why they *have* to come to dialysis because they aren't 'clean' enough. And the more they come the better they will begin to feel. Usually when patients first begin dialysis they feel really horrible and they think they are going to feel this terrible forever. Sometimes they feel so bad that they can't even begin to learn about their treatment. Then as they start correcting their anemia, lowering their uremia and getting their stamina up, they'll often say, 'Wow, I didn't realize how bad I felt.' Sometimes they start feeling the best that they've felt in two years. For many people, renal failure is slow and insidious, which is why folks won't realize just how long they've been sick until they rebound."

Do you have any success stories of patients who really made adjustments and followed your advice?

"The most memorable woman who comes to mind was a thirty-one-year-old African American woman who had nine children. This lady had such low self-esteem she barely made eye contact with me. Her phosphorus was off the charts."

Madeline explains that too much phosphorus—one of the impurities derived from the foods we eat—causes the bones to lose calcium. The calcium can move into the heart valves. Calcification of the heart can eventually lead to heart failure. Phosphorus molecules, unlike other impurities, are not as effectively removed from the bloodstream by the dialysis filter. This is why dialysis patients must take medications called binders. Binders literally bind or stick to phosphorous molecules, preventing them from entering the bloodstream and enabling them to exit the body via the bowels.

Madeline continues, "Initially when I told this young woman of the potential consequences of her dietary behavior she blew me off; she didn't think she would see me again. Here I was, this middle-aged white woman trying to tell her what to do. But I kept coming around to check on her. Eventually she asked me, 'Why you keep coming back?' I told her, 'You have nine kids. You are too young to kill yourself.' Slowly she began to engage with me. I would often ask, 'Do you have the money for your binders? Do you carry them with you?' Little by little her phosphorus declined. On the days she received her lab results she began looking for me. Watching her self-esteem grow was amazing. The day that she finally got her phosphorus to an acceptable level, all the nurses and technicians gathered round her to congratulate her on a job well done."

Typically what kind of training, education, or literature do dialysis patients receive in preparation of being dialyzed for the first time?

"Well, as I mentioned before, in reality a lot of people are introduced to dialysis after they are already on it. In a perfect world people would learn that they have high blood pressure or diabetes and they would take the steps necessary to try to prevent or postpone dialysis. Then if they did have to go on dialysis, there would be ample warning and time for them to get a permanent access. Ideally they wouldn't be initiated to dialysis in the hospital with a resident putting in a catheter. Rather, the nephrologist would say, 'Your GFR is getting down to 35%; let's put a fistula in you and if that doesn't work then a graft.' When someone has been followed for two or three years by a doctor and he or she comes into our clinic with a catheter I want to know why. My brother hasn't had a fistula put in yet, but I'm following his GFR levels and am frequently checking with his doctor as to when they are going to put it in."

What do you think is the most challenging for patients with a GFR of 15% or less who are new to dialysis?

"Coming to terms with the cards that they have been dealt. And sometimes they will do everything right and they will still have a setback and that is also very challenging. They might get sick, break a bone, be hospitalized and it just won't seem fair. Especially because they were doing everything right. And it isn't fair, but it wasn't fair that they got the disease in the first place. When they hit those bumps in the road they get frustrated and think 'How many times do I have to come in and get my access declotted?' or, 'How come I don't feel well enough to go to Angie's graduation?' Those are the times when it is the hardest for patients not to get the blues."

When it comes to educating people about dialysis what is the biggest challenge?

"I think with chronic patients the hardest thing is getting them to buy into taking care of themselves. For example, how do you make phosphorous management interesting? Someone who has been on dialysis for twenty years probably knows more about it than I do. A lot of times, it is not a lack of knowledge that keeps patients from following the guidelines. Rather, it is a lack of enthusiasm. Imagine someone who decides on January 1 to go on a diet and maintain a healthy lifestyle. Maybe he or she can do it for a week, but how will the person be doing come March? Or even come the second week in January? Getting folks to buy into their care and stick with it is the biggest challenge."

What do you like most about working with dialysis patients?

"People will say to me, 'How can you work at a dialysis clinic? Isn't it so depressing?' I don't think so. It really isn't. Overall people on dialysis do really well with that they've been dealt. Not one person there would be alive without dialysis—even if dialysis just means that they are able to play with their grandkids. This in itself can be a contribution so the parents can go to work. To me, working at a dialysis center is actually a glimpse of people at the very best they can be."

At the conversation's end Madeline mentions that she is grateful for the profession she has chosen. Having always held nurses in high esteem, she hopes more people will choose to become nurses. And she concludes, "Although some of us nurses have our warts, for most of us it still comes down to caring for the vulnerable." Madeline's particular choice of words is worth noting: caring for the vulnerable, not for the incapable. Something to ruminate on, as our tour of the suds factory is now complete.

Three

Dialysis Options

Choosing What Works Best for You

O NCE YOUR DOCTOR determines that you are indeed in need of—or will be in need of—dialysis or a transplant, then together you must decide which type of treatment, or which type of "modality" as it is often referred to by the medical community, will work best for you. In this chapter we will specifically focus on the variety of dialysis modalities that exist. In the next chapter we'll discuss at length the alternative modality: transplantation. You may already know that transplantation is your chosen route, but even so, it is very likely that you will be on dialysis for some amount of time before receiving a successful transplant. Or perhaps you are too sick to make any decisions about modalities when you first begin dialysis. That's OK. The good news is that you are not wedded to any particular dialysis modality. Even if you've already started on one kind of dialysis, you may opt to switch to another in the future. So whether you are awaiting a transplant or have already started a particular dialysis regime, we'd encourage you to read on.

These days there are actually several different kinds of dialysis, but each kind falls under one of two headings: peritoneal dialysis (PD) or hemodialysis. The goals of both types of dialysis are the same: again, to filter and remove the excess fluid and toxic impurities from your blood. Both types of dialysis can do the trick, but choosing the type is determined by each patient's unique needs as well as by each patient's responses to different types of treatments. Your particular medical history may limit your options and dictate your choice of modality. For example, someone who sustains scarring from a previous surgery to the abdomen may not be a candidate for peritoneal dialysis. Likewise, someone who suffers from poor venous circulation may not be a candidate for hemodialysis. And these two examples are but a drop in the ocean. We can't begin to capture all the medical circumstances that may dictate your choice of treatment, which is why, together with your doctor's guidance, you will determine which type of dialysis modality might work best for you. Our goal in this chapter is to provide you with insight into the types of dialysis available so that you can begin to ask your doctor the right questions.

First, two major differences between peritoneal dialysis and hemodialysis have to do with (1) who is in charge, and (2) where is it done. Peritoneal dialysis is carried out by you and can be done in the privacy of your home, workplace, or anywhere that meets sufficient standards of cleanliness. Hemodialysis can be done either at home, usually with the help of a partner, or, as is more common, in a center like the one we visited in the prior chapter, where nurses and technicians manage the procedure and where other patients dialyze alongside you at the same time.

Regardless of the kind of dialysis you choose, it will require work on your end—which is why being on dialysis should in some ways be thought of as a lifestyle choice as much as a medical procedure. It is for this reason that we strongly recommend that you take the time to research and identify the modality that can be best integrated into the rest of your normal world. When it comes to your health there are many things out of your control, but prohibitive medical issues notwithstanding, selecting your treatment of choice is one thing that you may very well influence.

The majority of the patients whose perspectives are shared throughout this book are on hemodialysis, and this majority is reflective of the dialysis population at large.[1] We ourselves are most familiar with hemodialysis because that is the modality that Daniel uses, and later in this chapter we will briefly examine its various types, including home hemodialysis. Let us focus first, however, on peritoneal dialysis and share the story of a patient for whom that modality works best.

We were delighted to meet Elena, a soft-spoken, yet feisty woman in her mid-fifties who has been coping with kidney failure for over three decades and who wholeheartedly sings the praises of peritoneal dialysis. When it comes to renal failure treatments, she has really done it all: hemodialysis for eight months, a transplant for nineteen years, followed by peritoneal for eight years, during which she sporadically returned to hemodialysis. When asked to rank each treatment in order of best to worst quality of life, without hesitation she said, "peritoneal, then transplant, then hemo." Surprised? We were. Perhaps you won't be after hearing her story.

Elena's Story: A Peritoneal Dialysis (PD) Patient's Perspective

Elena and Margie meet in a suburban public library. Elena kiddingly says that her house is a "mess." Margie finds this to be curious, because she assumes that, due to the risks of infection associated with peritoneal dialysis, one would need to be obsessively clean to achieve success. Elena sets Margie straight by explaining that the area where she performs her dialysis is quite clean, which is an absolute necessity of PD, but that the "mess" is everything around the periphery and really is a matter of clutter not dirt. By contrast, the small library room is the picture of order. Surrounded on all sides by shelves of books, Margie turns on her tape recorder and the two women get down to business.

Elena starts by explaining that while at work one day in 1972 she looked down and couldn't see her feet because her ankles were so swollen. She was twenty-four years old at the time. Soon after she was diagnosed with glomerulonephritis, a disease resulting from an inflammation of the kidney that destroys kidney tissue. Five and half years later, when she first began dialysis in 1978, she suffered from severe uremia and anemia. Because the pharmaceutical substitute for erythropoietin wasn't yet introduced and wouldn't be until the early 1990s, Elena was subjected to thirteen blood transfusions in eleven months. Elena was on hemodialysis for a relatively short period, eight months, before she received a kidney transplant from her brother.

What would you have liked to have learned when you first started dialysis?

"When I first developed renal failure I think I was too busy trying to survive to worry about learning anything. The second time I went on dialysis I would have liked to have heard about life after transplant. What I learned is that there is life after transplant—as it turns out, a pretty good one."

The first time you started on dialysis did you consider peritoneal dialysis?

"It wasn't an option then or, if it was, it wasn't discussed. When I started dialyzing, I was just lucky that Medicare paid for it. If I'd had to go on dialysis immediately, like when I had first noticed my swollen ankles in 1972, it wouldn't have been covered. The act that mandated Medicare coverage of dialysis didn't pass until 1973. Let me use a bit of Yiddish here—even a schlimazel [a luckless person] can have a bit of mazel [luck]—meaning I was terribly unlucky to get sick, but very lucky to get sick when I did. If I had gotten sick during my parents' generation we wouldn't even be having this conversation."

What advice would you give to someone who is new to hemodialysis?

"Think about peritoneal dialysis as soon as possible! I'm a peritoneal cheerleader so it is *really* hard for me to encourage anybody on hemodialysis. For some people hemodialysis is wonderful. They get the socialization with the other patients at the center, they get somebody taking care of them there in the event that something happens, but I'm too independent. I've fought too hard for my independence to choose hemodialysis. For me hemodialysis isn't a life, but it keeps me alive until I can weigh my choices and figure out what I want to do."

Elena goes on to tell Margie that after receiving her transplant she was able to finish school, return to work, enjoy an active social life, purchase her own home, and live independently. Her brother's kidney served her very well and lasted a few days shy of nineteen years. And as Elena says, "Considering when I was transplanted, it was quite a good run." But the years of immunosuppressant drugs had seemingly taken their toll. Designed to suppress the immune system so that her body would not reject her brother's kidney, these drugs also suppressed her body's ability to ward off ailments. While there is no evidence that the drugs were the direct cause, they did make it harder for her to fight the kidney cancer that she was diagnosed with. Desperate to save her kidney, Elena chose an out-of-network surgeon—the best physician for the job—to remove the cancerous tumors. At that point, she didn't know with certainty if her insurance company would pay for that particular physician's services, but as she tells Margie, "I would have sacrificed anything, sold my house if I had needed to and moved in with my sister, to try and save what I could." (The insurance company did pay, but Elena didn't learn this until the day before she went into surgery. She was fully prepared to go into debt to pay the costs herself.)

Unfortunately, a return to dialysis could not be thwarted. That fateful day, the on-call physician said to Elena, "Have you thought about peritoneal dialysis?" Elena said she had been told she wasn't a candidate. "That's ridiculous," replied the physician. Elena tells Margie that she now looks back on that meeting and feels incredibly fortunate to have been given such advice.

Describe peritoneal dialysis to me? What are your days like? What is your routine?

"I have a catheter inserted into my stomach wall, which exits my abdomen. It's a little plastic tube that sticks out of my belly. The catheter enables me to hook up a drain tube to the machine, also called the cycler. Everything goes in and out of that one tube. Unlike hemodialysis, you don't use any needles. The routine is this: you mask, wash, and then hook up to the machine. You introduce the solution into the abdomen. That is called the fill. You let it sit there for two hours. That is called the dwell and then you drain it. The entire process is called an exchange. When you drain the solution, you are removing the excess toxins and fluids from your body. The lining of your abdomen, the peritoneal cavity, filters the toxins and fluids from your blood."

Elena then explains that the two most common kinds of peritoneal dialysis are continuous ambulatory peritoneal dialysis (CAPD) and continuous cycling peritoneal dialysis (CCPD). With CAPD a person completes four or five exchanges throughout the day by hand, without the use of a machine. Dialysis fluid remains in the abdomen for four to six hours, allowing thirty to forty-five minutes to drain and fill. CCPD, Elena's dialysis of choice, uses a machine that continuously does the exchanges throughout the night. Sometimes when an individual is on CCPD, he or she might need to do one manual exchange during the day as well. Elena tells Margie that she completes four exchanges throughout the night. The machine drains, fills, then lets the solution dwell for almost two hours each time. Then at the end of the night, Elena receives one last fill. She then carries this fluid with her throughout the next day.

Do you sleep the whole ten hours that you are on the machine?

"I am up for the first drain, watching the news. I have a TV in my bedroom. I usually get about seven to eight hours of sleep. I am sometimes awakened by an alarm on the machine, and it will say low drain volume. That means that I'm not getting enough fluid out. For most people on CCPD, this is a rare occurrence. When it happens I hit the stop button to shut it up. Then I sit up or pace because I drain better when I'm upright. For that reason, I always try to get up and pace for the last drain. I have a plastic line that enables me to walk. And if need be, the line is long enough for me to walk to the bathroom."

Do you travel while on peritoneal dialysis?

"Not recently, but yes I have. I have traveled to North Carolina and six years ago I traveled to Israel. The flight to Israel was twelve hours plus I had a fourteen-hour layover in London. I had to get special permission to do this, but I asked my doctor, 'What do you want me to do?' He said, 'Dialyze before you leave for the airport and dialyze as soon as you arrive.' It was a very long time between dialyzing! I think the only reason he let me do this is because my labs were so good. My machine is twenty-five pounds. I put it in a suitcase which I carried onto the plane with me."

What are the advantages of peritoneal dialysis?

"First of all, like I said, I'm independent. Even though I have to do it every day, or should I say I *get* to do it every day, I can do it on *my* time. I don't have to start at 10 P.M. If I go out and I don't get home until 1 A.M., I just start then and dialyze until 11 A.M. the next day. Another big advantage is you can do it while you sleep. Another benefit about peritoneal dialysis is that it is portable. Obviously CAPD is the most portable; you can do it around town if you have to, but as I said, with CCPD I have taken my machine with me when I traveled. And I only need to visit the center once a month to meet with the doctor and have blood drawn for tests.

"Another huge advantage with peritoneal dialysis is that you don't get the ups and downs associated with hemodialysis. On hemodialysis you can feel these swings because you are growing uremic over a forty-eight-hour period and then you have the toxic wastes removed in just four hours. With peritoneal dialysis I'm constantly dialyzing so I never have those highs and lows. I'm on an even keel across the board. Now I don't cramp when I dialyze and I don't have to worry that I will have to jump out of bed because of cramps. When I was

on hemodialysis, if I got leg cramps, I couldn't even stand up and walk them off. With hemodialysis you are literally stuck in place."
Can you do peritoneal dialysis on an airplane?
"It has been done. There are people that do it in their cars. There are people who go camping and do it in their RVs. Would I do it? I don't think so. I'm too worried about the risk of infection."
Peritoneal dialysis patients can be at risk for infections externally at the site of the catheter as well as internally in the abdomen. Signs of infection include redness, swelling, soreness, and pus at the site of the catheter, which is usually surgically placed a few inches below one's belly button. An infection of the abdomen is called peritonitis. Most infections can be treated with antibiotics.
We've heard there is a high risk of infection with peritoneal dialysis; have you ever had an infection?
"I have had exactly one episode of peritonitis and I've been doing this for a little over eight years. When I got the infection they had to replace my peritoneal catheter, but first they wanted the abdomen to rest. No point in implanting a new catheter into an infected belly. So I went on hemodialysis for three months this summer. I would not profess to be the world's expert on cleanliness, and I manage. So I think others can do it too."
How do the dietary and liquid restrictions compare to hemodialysis?
"The diet restrictions are fewer. Not gone but less. The big thing is the phosphorous. I take binders and avoid dairy products because they are high in phosphorous. My potassium tends to be low, which is the opposite of patients on hemodialysis. I can either take a supplement or I can have a heck of a good time eating squash, tomatoes, bananas, and brussels sprouts."
As for the fluid restrictions Elena tells Margie there are none. Additionally she is able to control her blood pressure with the dialysate solutions she uses. There are different strengths of these solutions, meaning they have different amounts of dextrose (sugar): 1.5%, 2.5%, or 4.25%. The higher the concentration of dextrose, the more

fluid is removed. When Elena's blood pressure is low, she uses 1.5% solution. At times when it has been higher, she has used 2.5%. She does take her blood pressure both in the morning and at night, and she weighs herself twice daily in order to know how much liquid to remove though the course of the night.

Aside from the dietary restrictions, are there any other limitations with peritoneal dialysis?

"If I was younger and athletic there would be some limitations. You have to protect the abdomen. Also there is a great deal of debate, even among medical professionals, about swimming with a catheter. Some people believe swimming in a pool that is chlorinated is a sufficient protection against infection. Personally I have not gone swimming since I began PD. I am too concerned that I'll get an infection."

Certain precautions regarding water, bathing, and swimming need to be taken to protect peritoneal dialysis patients from infection. Unlike patients with temporary catheters in the neck or groin, peritoneal patients with catheters in their abdomens may shower, swim, or bathe. However, before showering or bathing, they need to place a protective plastic covering over the catheter. They may swim in chlorinated pools or the ocean, but may not swim in brackish or fresh water.

What is the biggest challenge with peritoneal dialysis?

"There are days when you say, I don't want to set up. I don't want to do this. But there are days on hemodialysis when you say the same. You get sick and tired of being sick and tired. You get sick of having to be reminded of it all the time. If all you do to manage a disease is pop a pill, that's no big deal. Dialysis is different. On hemodialysis you have to think to yourself, 'It's Monday; I have to be at the unit at four today.' Your time is constricted. That was what was so wonderful about going on peritoneal dialysis. All of a sudden I had the entire day back! My days weren't chopped up and at first they felt so long. But I quickly learned to love it."

What are the key success factors to living well with renal failure?
"I think that you have a choice. You can either roll with it, or you can curl up in a corner and wait to die. Now—since I'm not ready to wait to die, I roll with it. People say to me, 'How can you be on a machine for ten hours?' I say, 'You know what? There is no choice.' It's not that I'm making a choice. It's what I do. Period. Or people say, 'How can you be on this diet?' I say, 'You know what? I manage.' People don't get it. You have to take what you get and you have to live with what you get. The key to success is to be able to live with it without having it become the focus of your life. A lot of people do 'Oh poor me.' Or, they say, 'Why me?' The answer is, 'Why not.' "

Just as all good things must come to an end, so does Margie's meeting with Elena, and the women part with hugs and smiles like two old friends who have known each other for a long while.

Peritoneal Dialysis: Benefits and Drawbacks

Elena did an excellent job of laying out the hows and whys of peritoneal dialysis for a novice. To review and elaborate on her points, peritoneal dialysis (either CAPD or CCPD) may be a great modality for people who

- Want the flexibility to dialyze on their own schedule either every day at night for ten hours or every day for thirty to forty-five minutes at four- to six-hour intervals.

- Desire or at least be willing to assume a greater sense of ownership and control over their care.

- Are prepared to dialyze every day or night in order to have the added benefit of less uremia and fluid retention, which results in consistently better physiological well-being day to day.

- Have transportation limitations and perhaps can't easily get to a dialysis center three times weekly.

- Want to be independent from a hemodialysis unit—including its very rigid scheduling—with the exception of monthly visits for lab tests.

- Want to take care of themselves rather than passively let a technician hold the reins.

- Are frightened of needles or have veins that won't accommodate accesses.

- Want to worry less about how much they drink, and to have less stringent dietary restrictions.

- Are self-conscious about a visible access in the forearm and would prefer to have a catheter that can be concealed.

- Want the ability to travel with ease (especially those on CAPD) without having to dialyze at new and unknown dialysis centers.

- Want to be able to dialyze at home without having the help of a partner.

- Want to be able to dialyze at home but are worried that they can't learn how to do so—the training for peritoneal dialysis is easier than the training for home hemodialysis.

Peritoneal dialysis may also be a great modality for people who are willing and able to

- Conquer their intimidation and fear about taking on the role of home technician.

- Devote space in their home for the dialysis medical supplies and/or a cycler—imagine approximately the cubic space of a medium-sized closet or an average-sized washer and dryer.

- Overcome concerns that their family and other members of their household will have to be around them while they are dialyzing or that they will never feel like they can truly be *away* from dialysis.

- Diligently maintain a standard of cleanliness (washing, masking, etc.) that will protect the catheter against infection.

- Understand that in general there is increased risk of infection to the peritoneum (abdominal wall) or at the site of the catheter.

- Drain fluid before participating in sports or exercise and fill after.

- Carry a dextrose solution in the abdomen throughout the day and night, which can sometimes increase the size of the stomach and/or result in weight gain.

- If diabetic, monitor blood sugar levels even more carefully due to the sugar content of the solution that can increase blood sugar. Insulin may be added directly to the solution.

- Possibly shift to loose-fitting clothes that may be more comfortable given the placement of the catheter and a full belly.

- Forgo some self-consciousness and explore with a partner ways to have intercourse that are comfortable given the placement of the catheter in the lower abdomen.

- Move 2.5 and 5 liter bags of dialysis solution. This may not be ideal for someone who is weak or frail.

- Sleep while dialyzing, despite the noise that the machine may make throughout the night (specific to CCPD).

- Make the easy switch to manual exchanges in order to travel with ease or carry the machine if capable (specific to CCPD).

We also found it interesting to hear what many physicians and nurses had to say about the pluses and minuses of peritoneal dialysis:

- "Many people will shy away from peritoneal dialysis and say 'I can't do that!' My response is, 'Why can't you? You are smart enough to learn and we're going to teach you.'"

- "I try to encourage most young people to do peritoneal because the freedom for them is enormous. Plus peritoneal dialysis gives

them control, or at least more control over their life and their
disease so they feel like they are in charge. For many patients the
loss of control is traumatic and when they can recover some element of control, it's great."

• "Previously the perception was that peritoneal dialysis was for really good patients, ones who were highly motivated; now it is
  more commonly considered for all patients, including those with
  more disabilities."

• "I don't have hard data to support it, but I believe that people
  who take an active role in their care and their well-being are
  more vested and do better. As a result, I have a bias toward
  out-of-center modalities. The dialysis center is a very passive
  experience. It is easier for the technicians in the centers to have a
  passive patient than a patient who is going to come in and start
  asking questions or get involved. Even if you have a patient who
  wants to get involved, in many cases he or she is going to be dissuaded because of the nature of the system which needs to get
  patients in and out quickly and efficiently."

• "Do you have to be very clean on peritoneal dialysis? Well, you
  do and you don't. I've had blind people successfully do it, as well
  as folks who are very down and out socioeconomically. The most
  important thing is to have a good routine. You have to follow a
  rigid procedure and protocol for cleanliness. Most people can do
  it. I have found that most people who get an infection and were
  a bit sloppy before getting infected will self-correct after."

• In contrast, "For those who have difficulties with vision or impair-
  ments with motor skills or neuropathy, I try to steer them toward
  in-center hemodialysis unless they have a lot of support at home."

• "Most of my patients who do peritoneal dialysis, if they have to
  switch to hemodialysis, really don't like it. Several who have lost
  their peritoneal dialysis catheter for one reason or another are
  miserable on hemodialysis both physically and psychologically."

- "If I had to go on dialysis I would choose home hemodialysis as my modality, so I could do it whatever time of day I wanted to. I wouldn't have to drive to a clinic if the weather was bad. Peritoneal dialysis might be an easier modality for traveling, but I'm not sure if I'd want to go sloshing around with that much fluid in my abdomen. Plus, if you are on home hemodialysis, you don't have to do it every day."

Clearly there are numerous challenges and benefits associated with CAPD and CCPD. We hope that this section has been illuminating and that you now know more about peritoneal dialysis (we certainly do) than you did before hearing Elena's story. Now let's take a brief look at the other overarching dialysis modality—hemodialysis—and the specific types of hemodialysis and their benefits and drawbacks.

Spotlight on Hemodialysis: Continuing Your Search for the Best Dialysis Modality for You

When we spoke with the many in-center hemodialysis patients whose voices you'll hear throughout other chapters in this book, they often said that they had no interest in pursuing peritoneal dialysis. Nor would they want to do hemodialysis on their own, which is similar to in-center dialysis but usually requires a partner's assistance and entails having a dialyzer, needles, and the like in their home. Many said they did not want to burden themselves or their family members by having their medical condition, including an area devoted to machines and/or medical supplies, "in their faces" all the time. Sometimes patients simply didn't have the space in their homes to accommodate a dialysis setup. With regard to peritoneal dialysis, most didn't like the idea of "always dialyzing." In-center hemodialysis allowed them to come three days weekly and then, in theory, to be free from dialysis the other four days. With peritoneal dialysis, they perceived the seven-days-a-week routine to be a constant reminder that didn't grant them an "out of sight out of mind" escape. Many patients said they felt quite good when they left dialysis, and the fluid retention and buildup of impurities over a forty-eight- to seventy-two-hour period did not adversely affect them enough to warrant a change in modality.

In addition, most of these patients weren't particularly keen, or were downright nervous, about being in charge of a machine or their care at home. They preferred coming to a center and having a technician or nurse assume the burden of care and to be on hand in case of any emergencies. Some said they'd never really thought about peritoneal dialysis or home hemodialysis one way or the other. In-center hemodialysis is what they've been doing to date, and it was working for them well enough. Why change? Most told us that they have found a sense of community with the other patients whom they met in the chairs next to them or in the waiting room. Some patients mentioned forming friendly relationships with nurses and staff as well. Many described the people in the unit as a "family." Does having this sense of family make dialysis enjoyable? Well, that might be a stretch, but it certainly does make it more endurable.

Taking into account what we heard from these patients, in-center conventional hemodialysis may be an excellent modality for people who

- Want to dialyze only three times weekly and essentially leave dialysis when they walk out the door of the center.

- Want to, or are at the very least willing to, let trained professionals be responsible for managing the dialysis process.

- Enjoy the comfort and community of being around others who "get" what they are going through and are often in the same boat.

- Want the reassurance of knowing that medical assistance is easily available in the event of an emergency.

- Are physically or mentally incapable of caring for themselves on peritoneal dialysis or do not have a partner at home who can be with them during home hemodialysis sessions.

Hemodialysis may also be a good modality for people who are willing and able to

- Very carefully monitor their diet in order to minimize the ups and downs associated with uremia.

- Very carefully monitor their liquid intake in order to minimize stress on the heart, respiratory distress, and/or side effects associated with having to take off too much water during a session, such as cramping or flu-like symptoms.

- Adhere to the schedule that is determined by the dialysis center, make it a priority, and move any conflicting activities to another time (not always ideal for certain work and school schedules).

- Deal with the setbacks and losses of dialysis "family" members over time. An unavoidable fact is that many people who receive in-center treatment are dealing with complicating, life-threatening illnesses. Forming bonds, while emotionally uplifting, can also be sad and stressful when someone you see three times a week becomes worse, is hospitalized, or dies.

Aside from in-center conventional hemodialysis, there are other types such as home conventional, home short-daily, in-center nocturnal (nightly), and home nocturnal. Each of these is a variation on the basic in-center hemodialysis that we've described. The major differences between them are the location, frequency, duration of time, and time of day spent on the hemodialysis machine. In addition, as we've mentioned, home hemodialysis options require a training process, space in the home, an adequate utilities setup to run the hemodialysis machine, and usually the commitment of a partner who is present for every dialysis session. Having a partner may not always be a requirement, however; it is dependent on the policies of each clinic.

As we wrote this chapter, we realized that there are many factors for someone wanting to choose one dialysis modality over the other. One person might pass out at the sight of blood and needles while another might be a physician. One person might not think twice about drinking in moderation while another might really find it to be a challenge. One person might be an extremely light sleeper while another might be bordering on narcolepsy. One person might be a night security guard while another might be a daytime middle-school teacher. Pick any combination of these characteristics, give weights of importance to each, and you will likely arrive at very different dialysis modalities that seem to best fit a person's overall lifestyle and well-being. For example, one patient's personal modality advertisement might read like this: "Extremely needle phobic, mildly light sleeper who loves job as a school teacher. Has some free periods during the day, wants more control over her care and ability to drink more. Desperately seeks best dialysis modality." In this case, CAPD might be just the ticket.

But of course it is rarely this easy to arrive at a decision. What if we throw in the fact that this person lives in a tiny apartment without an inch of storage space? Well, then she may have to move to accommodate her peritoneal dialysis supplies or else kick her liquid-loving, needle-fearing ways and consider an in-center hemodialysis option. The bottom line: there is a give and take with every modality. Your job is to work with your doctor to find the one that gives the most and takes the least. Why make the effort? Because chances are it will profoundly impact the quality and longevity of your life. Once you've made your best-informed guess, then take the steps to make it happen.

For more information on the various forms of dialysis, please refer to the Helpful Resources section at the end of the book, ask your doctor, or contact a dialysis center near you for any literature or videos (which are usually produced by medical supply companies) that cover the different modality options.

Four

The Decision to Pursue
a Transplant

A s we've heard, dialysis is not the only option in dealing with
defunct kidneys. In fact, for many it is not even the *best* option.
Transplantation, agreed to be the preferable course of treatment for
the majority of patients, is a lofty subject and an entire book could
be spent on all that is involved before, during, and after a transplant.
This is not that book. This is a book about dialysis—how best to live
with, cope with, and adapt to it—an important subject even for the
sizable population awaiting a transplant. But given the interconnect-
edness of dialysis with transplantation in the treatment of kidney
failure, we would be shortsighted not to devote a chapter to the
overarching discussion of transplantation and the role of this treatment in the lives of dialysis patients. For one who chooses to pursue
transplantation, dialysis is still a necessary interim treatment until a
donor kidney becomes available. But who chooses transplantation
and for what reasons? Is it always an easy decision? Oftentimes yes,
but not always, and it is a choice that many dialysis patients grapple
with.

According to the Organ Procurement and Transplantation
Network (OPTN), the graft survival rates for kidney transplants
performed from 1997 to 2004 after one, three, and five years for
people between the ages of fifty and sixty-four years is approximately 91%, 81%, and 70% respectively.[1] These numbers reflect

the odds that a new kidney will be alive and functioning well within a recipient over these respective lengths of time post surgery. However, these statistics are a compilation of everyone who received a kidney transplant during those seven years, regardless of what year their surgery was performed. As you can imagine, the closer to the present day that one undergoes a transplant, the more likely the procedure is to succeed—due to ongoing advancements in transplantation medicine and care. Also, one's age and general state of health can improve one's odds that a kidney transplant will succeed. As an example of these improved odds, if you look at the survival success rates during the same period for recipients ages eighteen to thirty-four, the rates of success increase to 93%, 83%, and 72% in years one, three, and five.[2] Without a doubt, these numbers are very positive. In addition to the sheer success rates, physicians argue that for many, quality of life is improved and longevity of life is extended.

In this chapter, we describe what it might be like for someone with nonfunctioning kidney disease to opt for a transplant instead of a lifetime on dialysis. Through the course of gathering research for this book, we talked to nephrologists who weighed in as to who should seek transplants, dialysis patients who were eagerly awaiting transplants, and renal patients who had experienced successful transplants for many years but were now back on dialysis. But it was our interview with one gentleman who had successfully undergone a kidney/pancreas transplant three years prior that we felt best illuminated many of the issues involved with dialysis and transplantation. By sharing his insights here, we aim to provide an objective comparison of one man's life on dialysis versus his life with a transplant. We hope his story, in conjunction with the practical information that follows, will aid you in your decision-making process and, should you choose transplantation, realistically prepare you for some of the potential benefits and pitfalls involved.

Larry's Story, a Transplantation Patient's Perspective

It's a rainy, cool Sunday morning when Margie rings the doorbell of Larry's home. A middle-aged, medium-built, Caucasian gentleman with light brown hair opens the door and amicably welcomes her in. The two exchange small talk as Larry leads the way to a tiny room surrounded by windows—the room is just large enough for a table and two chairs. He inquires if this will be a good spot for the interview and awaits Margie's response before taking a seat. Before she can answer, he jokingly interjects that he is quite "the talker" and warns that Margie might have to rein him in. Usually Margie prefers to conduct in-home interviews in the kitchen, as she has found it to be a comfortable room that typically puts interviewees at ease. But both this nook and Larry exude warmth, and Margie knows that her kitchen strategy will not be necessary. She assures him it is an excellent spot, encourages him to talk freely, and begins to ask him about his life both before and after his successful kidney/pancreas transplant.

Larry explains that while he was diagnosed with diabetes and was insulin dependent at age twenty, he did not begin dialysis until three decades later. His renal failure came on very abruptly, surprising even his nephrologist by its rapid onset. Ultimately, a partner who was subbing for Larry's vacationing physician broke the news that Larry needed to start dialysis immediately. Larry tells Margie, "Frankly, when the word dialysis was mentioned, it was really very upsetting. I hadn't been adequately prepared for it at that point, because my doctor thought I had another year to go." When Larry's doctor returned from vacation, he reviewed the tests along with other behavioral indicators and actually gave Larry the option of putting dialysis off a bit longer. Larry emphatically recalls, "I told my doctor, you have *got* to be kidding me! I've been sitting here upset for two days and scared to death of this. I'm *not* leaving this hospital until I'm on dialysis. Let's just get it under way and start dealing with it.'"

What was your experience like when you first began dialysis?

"Oh God, it was awful. As my diabetes had grown increasingly complex, I'd become very matter-of-fact about my health problems. But dialysis all of a sudden shook me to my roots. It was frightening at first. I probably cried every night for a couple of weeks. Initially it was exhausting. I'd come out of there and just be wasted. Plus I maintained my full-time job. So it was both physically taxing and emotionally turbulent.

"Then one day about three weeks into it, after they'd removed most of the toxins that had built up in my system, I woke up and felt pretty good. Something changed, a switch clicked and I thought this isn't so bad. I mean it was never a *fun* experience but emotionally I changed, and I thought 'OK, I can do this. I'm going to get a transplant and until then I can handle this.' It was at that point I started taking very active, aggressive steps to get the transplant that I have now."

What do you wish someone had told you before you first went on dialysis?

"I wish I'd known about other ways that you could receive dialysis and had been more aggressive about pushing for myself. With hemodialysis I had an extremely difficult time sitting there and being idle for so long. I thought about bringing my laptop computer with me and doing work at the clinic but found that I'd be nodding off. My doctor told me that outside of the United States he'd seen clinics where they had stationary bikes for people to ride while they were dialyzed. I would have loved to have been able to get on a bicycle three times a week for some exercise."

How did you decide to have a transplant?

"In terms of how I decided, I don't think there was ever any question. It was just that I was going to do it. Even now I look back and realize that some of the things other people investigated—some of the implications and complexities of transplantation—I never even worried about. I just knew I wasn't going to contend with dialysis and diabetes for the rest of my life. I knew that being diabetic and on dialysis would be particularly difficult and I knew enough about diabetes to know that I faced a continued deterioration of my body. That just wasn't going to be an option."

Larry explains that both his nephrologist and endocrinologist were strong advocates for a transplant. He began checking which hospitals would be covered under his insurance plan and which of those hospitals his doctors recommended. After being on dialysis for two months, he attended a transplantation orientation designed to give patients, many of whom had traveled from all areas of the country, basic information so they could decide whether a transplant was of interest. Larry tells Margie, "I kept thinking 'I don't want information! All I want to know is where do I sign up?!' " At the end of the meeting he approached the hospital's Director of Transplantation and Pancreas/Kidney Transplant Coordinator, intending to ask just a few questions. An hour and a half later the three were still talking when Larry said, "OK, what is the next step?" The Transplant Coordinator responded, "You just took it." Apparently Larry had wholeheartedly demonstrated his commitment to transplantation.

He was then told that the screening process just to be put on the list would take six months. When Larry pressed about why it would take so long, he was told that the actual tests did not take that much time, but that the scheduling conflicts—working around people's jobs, family commitments, and even travel requirements for those who lived out-of-town—lengthened the process. Larry countered, "I've got vacation time in the bank. I'll give you *as much* of it as you want. I can stay in a hotel right by the hospital and you can just put me through all the paces. *Let's just do it.*" And they did. They sent him through all the physical and psychological evaluations fairly quickly. Five months after Larry began dialysis, he was officially put on the list.

How long until you received your transplant?

"I was fortunate to be at the right place at the right time. They told me to expect about a three- to four-year wait. I was in it for the long haul. I was ready to just hunker down and stay healthy and wait. One day my transplant coordinator called and said, 'Things have been moving more quickly than expected and you are getting close to the top of the list in your blood group.' My first call was about three months after I was listed. It was a false alarm, meaning that the kidney turned out not to be usable for one reason or another. I had two false alarms before I got my transplant on March 20. It was ten months after I had started dialysis."

Larry describes those ten months as a time when he lived his life from day to day as well as he could. Forced to cut down on certain activities due to his lowered energy levels, he quit coaching his kids' sports teams. He couldn't maintain that level of activity as well as dialyze and work full time. But he tells Margie, "I had learned from being a diabetic all those years that you do what you need to do to get from one day to the next. I always thought dialysis was part of a larger process and it was getting me to the next step. I never saw dialysis as an end stage. I kept thinking, 'Put one foot in front of the other every day. Go to dialysis and then come home. Yeah, it's not fun but it is leading you to something else in three years and then you will be done.'"

While waiting, Larry was also preparing to switch to a form of home hemodialysis. With it, he was looking forward to having a more normal diet, drinking more, reducing his lethargy, and cutting down on his cramping and blood pressure fluxes. Larry was in the midst of undergoing training at a nearby hospital and was awaiting the arrival of his own home machine when he got called for his transplant.

Did you do anything physically or mentally to prepare for your transplant?

"Physically, I just tried to be active because I wanted to be as healthy as possible going into it. Mentally, I don't recall having any worries. I didn't pay attention to some of the risks involved. There was never any question or hesitation in my mind if this was the right thing to do. I was fully prepared, motivated and ready to do it."

What emotions did you experience when the call came?

"When the call came and it was the real thing my wife became very emotional. I, on the other hand, was in a take-charge mode. My wife was getting upset and I told her to stop. I felt like I was going into battle. I was driving to the transplant center dictating to my wife things that needed be done: my boss needed to be called, co-workers needed to be given files, family members needed to be contacted. That was my way of dealing with it. I became stone cold—not fearful, just very matter of fact. If there were any emotions there I wasn't aware of them. I was just hoping for the best.

"I now know that there were many things to be afraid of—things that I don't think I was prepared for, and I'm just as happy that I wasn't. I encountered some very challenging and somewhat awful things. But even knowing what I know now I would *never* have made a different decision."

According to Larry, he was a "poster child" for the transplant; going into it and the actual seven-hour surgery went as well as it could. Both organs—the kidney and the pancreas—started functioning before they stitched him back up. Larry recalls waking up and hearing from a resident that he'd done great. Larry smiles and tells Margie, "I told the resident the first thing I wanted to do on my way home from the hospital was stop by my son's favorite ice cream parlor for a hot-fudge sundae and the second was to pick up a six-pack of Guinness stout. I also remember asking him if I'd be able to play the piano when I went home. He said, 'Sure, you'll be able to do anything you want.' And I said, 'Great because I've never been able to play the piano before!' "

Unfortunately, that was the last joke Larry would make for some time. Moments later, his throat began to fill with blood and his lungs began to lose oxygen. Then Larry's heart stopped. Or as he tells Margie, "I died on the table. They had to use the paddles on me three times to restart my heart." Larry later learned that when the doctors had withdrawn his breathing tube, an edge of the tube had caught on some soft tissue, cutting and filling his throat and then his lungs with blood. Looking back on the scare, he shrugs and says, "It was a fluke. Just one of those things. It happens." Larry then spent three days in intensive care during which he remembers telling his wife that he was having second thoughts as to whether the transplant was the right thing to do. Larry tells Margie, "My wife was *crushed.* All I knew was I felt miserable. It was a horrible process and a pretty startling experience."

After two weeks in the hospital, a week longer than the norm, Larry returned home in April and went back to work part-time in July. While other transplant recipients have been known to return to work as early as three weeks post surgery, Larry tells Margie that he was particularly weak from not eating due to the complications with his throat. "I wanted to ease back into work slowly and I'm so glad that I did. It was exhausting at that point."

Did you urinate right away? Were there any other immediate, noticeable physical differences?

"I did start urinating while I was still in the hospital. If you don't, there is the looming threat that at some point they'll have to put a tube in you. That was enough of a threat that I kept thinking 'I'll work on it!' "

Larry explains that with his new pancreas he no longer has to take insulin or test his blood sugar. "I thought it would be a very difficult transition having been an obsessive insulin-dependent diabetic, testing myself seven to eight times daily, keeping meticulous reports on my blood sugar. Little did I know! I never looked back. One day I woke up and realized I hadn't tested my blood sugar for two months and hadn't even thought about it! It was amazing."

At what point did you relax knowing that the organs were working?

"Oh it took awhile. I assumed that based on the number of times you had to go in and be tested if something wasn't working they would let you know quickly. My doctors couldn't have been more delighted with the outcome. Everything was working the way they wanted it to, and I trusted the doctors implicitly.

"I think there is always some question about whether the organs are working the way they are supposed to. I know from the way that I feel that they are working, but I do know there are things that go wrong. It's amazing how much maintenance and activity is involved once you've received the transplant. Sometimes symptoms arise and I wonder, 'Is this a rejection?' One morning about a year ago I was feeling miserable. I took my blood pressure. It was soaring. My blood sugar was too. I thought, 'I'm going into acute rejection.' It was really very frightening."

As it turns out Larry had contracted a rare kidney virus, which the doctors were able to get under control and continue to monitor over time. He tells Margie that he has noticed from visiting online chat forums that many transplant recipients refuse to worry about rejection. They claim that worry would defeat the purpose of getting the transplant in the first place, which was to lead a normal life. However, Larry remains very aware of the kidney infection.

Are there other collective thoughts that you hear transplant recipients emphasize?

"I think there is an unrealistic expectation that people have going into a transplant that can lead to a sense of disappointment and discouragement that life isn't perfect afterward. Folks who get kidney/pancreas transplants often complain that things aren't perfect. It is true. Even though your organs work, things aren't perfect. There are various viruses that you can contract. Regularly, you have to get your blood tested and occasionally you may have unexplained increases in your creatinine levels, which can be unnerving. I still occasionally am anemic and will need to get a shot to boost my red blood cells. Without doing much of anything, I somehow ended up with a stress fracture in my leg. Just like dialysis patients, transplantation patients are often still dealing with the increased brittleness of their bones. Now, one of the immunosuppressant medications that I take to protect my new organs prevents my bones from healing quickly, so the fracture took about seven months to heal."

What is your medication regime?

At this point Larry goes into the next room and returns with what looks like a bucket one would use for cleaning supplies—a small donut with the handle in the middle—but instead of polishes and sanitizers it is filled with medicine bottles of all sizes. "These are my morning meds," he says pointing to one side of the bucket. "These are my afternoon meds. Luckily my health insurance covers this. I'm getting about $18,000 of medications for about $30 a month. I have medications that keep my body from rejecting the organs, medications for migraines, medications for the kidney virus, medications for blood pressure, and medications for my bones. The number of medications has slowly grown as time has gone on. It is an interesting struggle to remember what to take."

Larry continues to regale Margie by pointing out a medication that he takes only on Mondays and Fridays, then a medication that he takes different doses of every other day, yet another he takes on Mondays, Wednesdays, and Fridays. "I have to be obsessive about keeping track of them. They are organized in a progression of what to take when. If anyone touches them I would know."

What do you consider the biggest drawbacks of the transplants?

"The drawback is my life has gotten more complicated in ways that I'd never expected. I complained recently to my doctor about how much goes into monitoring and managing these organs, the number of lab tests that I have to do, the medications that I have to take for the virus, the stress fracture. To this my doctor replied, 'Everything in medicine has costs and benefits.' I think I've experienced them all. Now that I have a transplant, life is not golden. I still have things going on in my body that need special attention. I'm a very expensive, high-maintenance individual."

What do you consider the biggest benefits of the transplants? What has changed?

"*Everything.* Everything has changed. First of all and most important, *it has normalized my life.* I no longer am dealing with two life-threatening conditions that were going to get progressively worse. The transplants have eliminated them for now. I certainly have a life in front of me, which is somewhat difficult to get used to. I just expected that I was going to die young. My father died young from complications from diabetes so I always thought I would too. I've got to adjust and actually plan for a future, now that I've got a life and, God willing, these organs will last for some time."

Now that you've done both dialysis and transplantation, what is your view of dialysis?

"Awful. I had sessions when I'd cramp horribly or I'd come home and have dinner and have stomach cramps. Or I'd have sessions when my blood pressure would drop and they'd have to treat me in an urgent way. Dialysis is life prolonging and maintaining, but I found it to be an awful experience to endure."

What advice would you give to someone who is waiting for a transplant?

"My first recommendation is get comfortable with the Internet. Get as much information as you can so you are going into it as well educated as you can be. Second, search out a support group. There are even online groups that are useful for sharing information and raising issues that you may have. Information is critical for people who need to take some control of their life.

"The other recommendation is maintain a sense of humor about all of this! It is deathly serious but my sense of humor has gotten me through an awful lot. To this day my doctor thought I was kidding about wanting to take my kidney home with me. As it turns out they don't take the old ones out; they just find spots for the new ones.

I had a vision of taking slices of my kidney and pressing them into slides and giving my friends coffee cups with a slide of the kidney that said 'Larry went to the hospital and all he got me was this damn piece of kidney.' People thought that was really sick. I thought it was wonderful sick! There *has got to be* a place to laugh."

Despite the weightiness of the subject matter Larry has been funny, energetic, and charming throughout the interview, which, without Margie even noticing, evolved from its intended one hour to two. Throughout their conversation it has been obvious to Margie that even with its massive hardships and trials, Larry *loves* life. She thanks him for his candor and willingness to share his story. Before leaving Margie asks to stop in the restroom and then admits to Larry that ever since Daniel went on dialysis, hearing herself or anyone "go" has taken on a whole new meaning. Now hearing that sound is like music to her ears. It is the sound of a healthy kidney. Larry understands this admission and laughs in agreement.

Transplantation: The Alternative to Dialysis

Who Is a Good Fit for Transplantation?

Many times, when we are young and trying to make a decision, we are advised to take a piece of paper, fold it in half, and on one side write down all the positives of the decision and on the other, all the negatives. As we heard from Larry, he has lived the lists—on both sides of the page—but knowing what he knows now he wouldn't have done anything differently. Upon hearing his story, we immediately recognized that he was an extremely energetic, animated individual who, in the prime of his life, clearly would have struggled enormously with the idleness involved with dialysis. He was so averse to inactivity that he even wanted to get on a bike and work out while his blood was being cleaned. Larry's nephrologist and transplantation surgeon deemed him an ideal candidate for transplantation. But what does that mean exactly? Who is an ideal candidate? Who is simply a good candidate? Who will be a long shot for making the list?

First, we'd recommend that you should at least have the conversation with your doctor about whether transplantation would make sense for you given your age and physical condition. As the best resource for making this determination, your doctor will steer you toward the treatment that will likely give you the best potential outcome in terms of quality of life and longevity. If advised by your nephrologist to pursue transplantation, you will be referred to a transplant center to be evaluated and screened. The transplant medical team will ultimately decide based on physical, social, and psychological factors whether you are an acceptable candidate.

In meeting and interviewing several nephrologists, we learned that all were strong proponents of transplantation but acknowledged that they recommend it on an individualized basis. All agreed that for those who fall into the category of "good to ideal candidate," it is the best way for patients to recover the closest resemblance to a normal life and to increase their life expectancy as well.

So who is considered a good to ideal candidate? Responses varied from doctor to doctor. One physician told us that he tries to refer all of his patients who can sustain the operation, which is a fairly straightforward surgical procedure to the abdomen. According to him, transplantation itself is not a big surgery; it is the manipulation of the immune system following the transplant and the heavy medical regime that can be more difficult than the procedure itself. Another physician said that most patients with nonfunctioning kidneys should at one point in their lives have a transplant, although he acknowledged that it gets trickier for older patients who are contending with additional life-threatening diseases. What is not crystal clear is where the line falls between young and old.

Of the doctors we spoke with, all said that patients under the age of fifty-five are considered young and more ideal candidates for transplantation than patients who are older. For those who are fifty-five and older, by each additional year, the determinants of candidacy become a bit grayer and more subjective depending on the physical and emotional health of the individual. That is when you have to begin to weigh the costs versus the benefits more carefully. According to OPTN in 2005, of the 16,477 people who received kidney transplants, 8,132 were under the age of fifty, 6,166 were between the ages of fifty and sixty-four, and 2,179 were over sixty-five.[3] But far and away the majority of people living with kidney failure are over the age of forty-five. According to the 2005 U.S. Renal Data System Annual Report, there are approximately five people over the age of forty-five living on dialysis for every one person under the age of forty-five living on dialysis.[4] When you put these facts together, you can see that with an increase in age comes a decrease in the numbers of transplants. But these numbers also emphasize that there is no hard and fast rule regarding age and that a significant number of older individuals in their fifties and sixties have successfully undergone transplants.

Another physician explained that his approach to treatment of patients with renal failure is like piecing together a jigsaw puzzle where each piece is a type of life extender. As he sees it, most renal patients are likely to have a finite time that they can live on dialysis: perhaps twenty to thirty-five years, depending on the individual. And there is likely a finite time that most transplanted kidneys will probably last: approximately ten to thirty years, again depending on the individual. So piecing together these life extenders for a young person with nonfunctioning kidney disease might entail a specific sequence of three pieces: five years on dialysis, thirty with a transplant, and then another twenty back on dialysis. This is just an example, but in this physician's mind, this comprehensive approach toward treating nonfunctioning kidney disease pieces together a life that otherwise would not be lived. Elena whom we met in the prior chapter is a living example of such an approach.

Consistent with this holistic approach to life extension and longevity, this same doctor admitted that he discourages patients in their sixties or seventies who are living well on dialysis from pursuing a transplant. He speculated that his approach may not coincide with that of the majority of his peers. But in his opinion, for those who are doing well on dialysis there is not a clear upside to transplantation in terms of longevity while there is a downside in terms of increased risks of complications. In his estimation, patients who are tolerating dialysis well and are maintaining a good quality of life know what they have on dialysis. However, they don't know what they will have with a transplant. As an example, Daniel went on dialysis at the age of sixty-nine after undergoing an elective triple bypass surgery prompted by chest pain. Over the latter half of his life, Daniel's track record was fair in terms of recovering complication-free from surgeries. Even his bypass had led to additional complications, including a small stroke and his kidney failure. After adjusting to life on dialysis, he considered transplantation but opted to stick with what he knew was working. At age sixty-nine, he was willing to trade the discomforts of dialysis for the added comfort of knowing, for the most part, what he was dealing with and what was working fairly well for him.

Who else might not be considered to be among the best candidates? Patients with severe heart disease, lung disease, obesity, or a host of other complicating, life-threatening diseases may be more likely to be dissuaded from or rejected for transplantation. But remember, each person is assessed as an individual by a nephrologist. Regardless of your age or physical disposition, if you really feel that transplantation is right for you, talk to your doctor.

Are there individuals who are good candidates but who choose not to pursue transplantation? Yes, there are some individuals who for one reason or another make this choice. Elena benefited tremendously during her lifetime from a transplant. She has been told that she is immunologically favored for another successful transplant because she did so well with the first one. Yet despite this positive prognosis, she has decided not to pursue a transplant. Why? Having suffered from cataracts, diabetes, and high blood pressure—all likely side effects of the immunosuppressants—and given her current success with peritoneal dialyis, she is hesitant to put her body through that again. Or as she says, she is "tired of rocking boats."

Transplantation for Dialysis Patients: A Cost-Benefit Analysis

As we heard from Elena and Larry, there are always costs and benefits to every option in medicine. The goal is to choose the better option. Looking at Larry's scenario, the benefits of dialysis were these: it extended his life, significantly improved his emotional and physical health by removing the toxins in his body, and enabled him to get a transplant. Alternatively, the costs were that he couldn't stand the idleness of visiting a center three times weekly; he had to endure cramping, drops in blood pressure, and overall exhaustion; and he was limited to very stringent dietary/liquid restrictions.

On the flip side, the benefits of transplantation were that he was able to regain a sense of normalcy; he no longer had to follow what he described as a "cardboard" diet; he no longer had to go to dialysis (which he despised) three days weekly and deal with the idleness and the physical side effects like exhaustion and cramping; he no longer was dealing with diabetes, which would have increasingly debilitated his body; and for the first time in his life he could imagine living a long life rather than dying young. Obviously these were no small benefits.

The costs of the transplantation were that he now has to maintain a rigorous and expensive medicinal regime and endure ongoing tests to monitor the health of the transplanted organs. He faced a serious life-threatening complication from the surgical procedure and encountered alternative medical problems such as the kidney infection and the slow-healing stress fracture.

We see from Larry that while one solution was clearly better for him than the other, neither was perfect. And as one physician who was a proponent of transplantation told us, "Getting a transplant is not like going back to having your own kidney and life the way it used to be. If people have expectations that aren't realized, it can be a very difficult transition for them." Or as Elena said, "People need to understand that a transplant is a treatment. It is not a cure and it is not a panacea either. There is not a cure for kidney failure. There are only treatments."

Larry's medicinal regime is representative of what is required post transplantation for the life of the organ. Human immune systems are designed to protect our bodies against foreign invaders such as bacteria, viruses, or foreign objects. This would include a healthy donated kidney. The immune system's natural response is to produce antibodies that would try to attack the kidney. Therefore, to protect a transplanted organ, one must take immunosuppressants, drugs that literally suppress the immune system from reacting as it naturally would. Immunosuppressents must be taken in perpetuity for the life of the organ. Even missing one dose of a drug can be detrimental to the health of the transplanted kidney.

For many, simply taking the pills all the time is what gets to be the biggest challenge, especially when they are feeling well. One doctor told us his patients will at times question why they still need them if they are feeling great. His answer, "Taking your medications is like following a religion when you do something solely because God says so. You have to have that kind of fervor and attention to it day in and day out."

Here is the good news: over time the medical and pharmaceutical industries have improved the drug therapies used to sustain donated organs. In the 1970s, patients would get huge doses of drugs and often fall very ill from infections, sometimes requiring additional surgeries. Now the field of transplantation has become better at managing and getting people and their grafts (kidneys) through the first year, also known as the acute rejection stage.[5] As Elena and Larry both point out, there are serious side effects associated with taking these medications—including but not limited to bone fractures, diabetes, infections, and cancers; these are very real possibilities that will affect some people more than others. However, there are also more choices of medicines available now, so there are more options for treating the side effects in a reasonable way. We recommend that you discuss all the potential side effects with your physician.

Other costs that need to be taken into consideration and planned for are monetary costs of screening and preparing for transplantation, costs of the surgery, as well as ongoing costs of the medications after the transplant. Larry was fortunate to have excellent health insurance through his job that covered both the costs of his transplant and his current prescription drugs. Many folks will find that they need to create a financial plan that will often draw from multiple resources to cover all the costs associated with transplantation.

There are many resources and organizations available to help you with financial planning and aid, several of which we've listed in the resource section at the end of the book, and your transplant center should have staff to assist you with planning as well. Sometimes obtaining money from savings, by fund-raising, or from charitable organizations will be necessary to ensure that you can purchase the medicines required to keep a donated kidney healthy.

For individuals concerned about the financial burden, one doctor advised, "Don't over-agonize about it. For patients who want and need their life back, where transplantation is the best option, they'll likely be able to work afterward and will do better in many ways. Finances should not become such an overwhelming issue that they prevent someone from being evaluated for a transplant."

The same physician told us of a patient who had undergone a successful transplant but who after three years was no longer covered for the costs of his transplantation drugs under the Medicare prescription drug benefits. The patient had two young kids and a good job, but without the prior Medicare coverage he couldn't sustain thousands of dollars in pharmaceutical bills. He was ashamed that he couldn't pay for the medications, so he stopped taking them and didn't tell anyone. He didn't want to admit that he was struggling. Without the medications, a person may remain symptom free for days, weeks, or even months, but a silent, certain rejection of the kidney begins taking place immediately. A few months later his wife found out and said, "No way! You have to call the doctor this minute!" The doctor scrambled around, pulled some samples of medications together, and worked to secure financial aid for the gentleman in need. The moral of this story: do not let your pride get in your way, plan ahead, and ask for help if you need it. Sometimes it takes time and paperwork, but there are resources available to assist with transplantation costs.

Transplantation: It Takes Two to Tango

We've talked about determining who is best suited for a transplant and some of the inherent costs and benefits of the procedure, but what about the kidneys themselves? Where do they come from and what are the costs and benefits to the donors?

The nice thing about kidneys is that most of us are born with two but we only need one to live a normal life. This means that transplanted kidneys can come from both living and deceased donors. In 2005, according to OPTN, of the 16,477 transplants that were performed, 9,914 kidneys came from a deceased donor while 6,563 came from a living donor.[6] In September 2006, there were 67,655 individuals cited by the OPTN as waiting list candidates for a kidney transplant.[7] Unfortunately these combined numbers definitively illustrate that there is a shortage of organs. The good news is that in 1990 only 22% of all donations came from living donors, but in 2005, approximately 40% came from living donors.[8] This means that the donor pool is on the rise.

Traditionally, living kidney donors would have to recover from a four- to eight-inch incision made in their lower back to remove one of their kidneys. A recently developed alternative procedure, laparoscopic surgery, enables doctors in some cases to retrieve the donated kidney through a few smaller incisions. This can lead to a faster and less painful recovery for the donor. Nonrelated living donors are also on the rise—meaning that increasing rates of organs are coming from individuals not related to the patients. Some hospitals are now even successfully performing concurrent kidney swaps in which, as an example, two families have an individual who needs a kidney, each has an individual willing to donate, neither donor is a match for his or her own family member in need, but *is* a match for the other donor's family member. With the introduction of creative new techniques and procedures such as these and others, we will likely see the pool of potential living donors continue to increase.

This book is written for dialysis patients and their families. If you fall into the second category, you may be thinking about becoming a living donor. You would be well served to think through the decision carefully. Be sure that you are doing it willingly and without pressure from your loved one or other family members. You don't want to find yourself resentful or feeling bullied into undergoing surgery. As with any straightforward surgery, there are health risks involved. The most common risks are infection and bleeding. There are also costs involved in the procedure. Depending on your family member's insurance, your costs may be covered by the recipient's insurance. However, there may be incidentals such as airfare, hotel stays, food, and loss of wages that may not be covered. You and your family member should research what will or will not be covered.

If ultimately you decide you wish to be a donor, you will be required to undergo a number of tests to determine whether your kidney is a match. Additionally there will be a psychological assessment to ensure that you are making a healthy, well-thought-through decision and that you are emotionally prepared for the possibility that, despite your best efforts, the recipient of your kidney may experience an acute or longer term rejection of your organ. There are significant benefits to receiving a kidney from a living donor versus a deceased donor. The recipient can schedule the procedure and begin taking immunosuppressant medications in advance, which helps reduce the risk of rejection. Typically, the success rate is higher and anti-rejection rates are lower among blood relatives whose tissues match. And the primary benefit to you as a donor is a sense of pride and contentment in knowing that you gave your loved one, or even a stranger, the greatest gift possible: independence from dialysis, a heightened sense of normalcy, and an improved quality of life.

There is a great deal of information available about transplantation, and because we are able to provide only a sliver of this content here, we recommend that you visit the book's resource section to find out where you can learn more. Our goal in this chapter was to describe broadly what transplantation involves and where it fits in the life of a dialysis patient. By sharing Larry's struggles and celebrations, we aimed to give you insight into many of the issues you should be discussing with your doctors. And by providing you with basic, useful information, we hoped to empower you to move forward with added strength and confidence in the health care decisions you make now and in the future. We also hope that, like Larry, you are able to embrace life and your decisions regarding how best to prolong and live it to the fullest. And remember, don't forget to laugh.

Five

The "K-Team"

Working with Dialysis Professionals

O NCE DIALYSIS IS introduced into your life, so are numerous individuals whom you had probably never wished to meet! They are the men and women who, with your active participation, will take a comprehensive, team approach to providing medical care for you while you are on dialysis.

While your access may be considered your lifeline, the doctors, nurses, dieticians, social workers, and technicians with whom you will interact could be coined your A-team, or perhaps more appropriately, your K (as in kidney) team. Each K-team member will play a vital role in your ongoing care. In this chapter, we will discuss how best to navigate, understand, thank, question, influence, co-exist, and in general, work with these individuals to achieve the best possible outcome. We define the best possible outcome as a very self-serving one: it is not to be the most popular, most loved, or most passive patient, but rather it is to be the patient who receives the best possible care at any given time. Understanding the strengths, weaknesses, roles, and perspectives of each member on your K-team will give you a leg up on achieving this goal. In this chapter we will provide helpful tips and insights that we and others have gleaned along the way when working with these critical members of our team.

First, though, let's hear an alternative perspective on dialysis from a pivotal member of the team, a nephrologist. Throughout our research we met with several nephrologists whose insights are shared intermittently in this book, but in the case of Jack we found his interview with Susan spoke best to the unique dynamic of the relationship between a doctor and a chronically ill patient. After weeks of phone and e-mail tag, Susan was able to secure an hour on Jack's calendar. Like most nephrologists, his time was in short supply. Despite this, he was more than willing to meet with her once his schedule permitted.

Jack's Story, a Nephrologist's Perspective

The day of the interview, Susan arrives at a bustling dialysis clinic at ten A.M. The receptionist ushers her through the doors of the waiting room and introduces her to a very tall man who like the stereotypical doctor stands beside a patient, reading and jotting notes on pages of paper attached to a clipboard. Jack shakes Susan's hand warmly and directs her to a small office off to the side of the clinic. He explains that he just needs to finish up with the patient and will be with her momentarily. True to his word, he does not make her wait long. Entering the office with a burst of energy, Jack takes a seat across from Susan and immediately begins answering her questions.

Jack tells Susan that he has been practicing nephrology for over fifteen years. When he first started in the field, he was more focused on research and teaching, but in time his focus shifted to actual patient care and treatment. He is now a member of a sizable nephrology practice that services two dialysis clinics and approximately 250 dialysis patients. Jack explains that one doctor from the practice is at each clinic every day. This schedule enables each patient to see a doctor every week to ten days and each doctor to see about eighty patients a week. Obviously the physicians' caseloads are heavy and their time is in demand. But Jack tells Susan that he and his colleagues maintain consistency with their shifts, so that the patients at the clinics will typically see the same physicians in the practice. "That way," he says, "we get to know the patients, their family members, who they are, their religious beliefs, what matters to them. With time, we begin to know the patients well and can provide a better level of continuity of care."

Jack explains that this continuity is especially beneficial if a patient is hospitalized. When a patient has a setback and arrives in the hospital after a medical event—or as Jack calls it, "an episode of care"—he or she is usually more debilitated and vulnerable than usual. And Jack concludes, "During these times it is very valuable to have a physician who is very familiar with that patient and his or her history. That way, the patient doesn't have to re-tell his or her whole story. Much of modern health care isn't built for that type of continuity, but it is especially important when someone has a chronic disease."

As a physician how do you define someone who is living well on dialysis?

"Doctors look at the lab tests and blood pressure and this and that. Of course, that is part of it. We need to know that the treatment is working as intended. But that's not the whole deal. We need to ask, what really matters to the patients? Are they doing the things in life that they like to do? Are they feeling relatively well at home? Are they having a reasonable level of activity? Are they enjoying their family? Those are clearly questions for the patients. Sometimes, I look at the lab tests and blood work and say, 'You are doing great!' and then I look down at the patient and clearly he or she is not. How that person is *really* doing is what you begin to understand as you talk to the patient and to the family. And, as you get to know them, they begin to trust you. They will confide in you. They may even confide in you if they are reflecting on whether or not to continue dialysis. But to answer your question—to me it means the person is actually feeling like 'I'm OK. This is good. I can live like this. Dialysis is worth it.' "

What percentage of dialysis patients that you see do you think are doing well—by your definition—on dialysis?

"It is tough to put your perspective on someone else's existence. I always tell my patients, this road you go alone. I call it the cliff. They look. They stare over the side and they decide if they want to do this. It is life changing for everyone. Probably 80% of the patients are satisfied that they are doing better and reasonably well on dialysis. I think a good 20% struggle. Some of the struggle is because other diseases they are coping with are collapsing in on them."

Jack explains to Susan that for many patients, especially those with diabetes, kidney disease is just one complication of many. Many times complications associated with diabetes—amputations, nerve damage, loss of vision, and vascular insufficiencies—all tend to hit at the same time. Jack tells Susan that often patients who are contending with many of these complications at once are on dialysis but are not satisfied with their quality of life. In these cases Jacks says, "The patients simply exist with the hope that things will get better."

What is the most challenging for patients who are new to dialysis and their families?

"The first few weeks or months can be difficult until they settle into a routine. Sometimes they get sick and get sent back into the hospital, then they need to have their accesses built, then they have a problem with their accesses and need to get them rebuilt; meanwhile they've got a catheter that isn't working well and they need a new one and everybody is thinking 'What the heck is going on!?' But what they need to understand and what is difficult for them to understand is that the beginning is rarely representative of what life on dialysis will be like. Trying to understand and see through all this turmoil can be very hard. Patients and families manage and get through it, but these rough starts add to their fears and worries. At the same time they are seeing all the other patients around them and they are thinking 'Oh my God what is this? Is this really my life?' "

What are common questions that patients and family members will ask you when they first begin dialysis?

"Sometimes they don't ask a lot of questions. You have to go after them to ask you questions. They will ask if dialysis is going to hurt. They won't always understand that dialysis doesn't make the kidneys better and that it doesn't cure them. They will ask how long until they don't have to do dialysis anymore. Most often patients will have that deer-in-the-headlights look."

Is it challenging for you to influence patients to manage their diet and liquids?

"Yes, it is a huge challenge. We are so used to doing what we want. This is our culture. There is food all around us. All our friends are eating. When you are on dialysis, you can't walk around with a "Big Gulp" like you used to, but some patients do! We are in this constant battle with some patients. They come in, we remove fluids, they feel sick and they think that dialysis is killing them. What I have to make them understand is that if they were more careful, they would feel better. My approach when this happens is to say, 'Do this for two weeks and you will see a difference. Just two weeks.' Some people figure it out and some never do."

Have you had patients who have ultimately chosen to stop dialysis?

"Yes. Not many. It is a difficult and enormous decision for someone to make. It has to be a very thoughtful decision. For example, most patients can't think clearly or thoughtfully right after they've had coronary bypass surgery. They may be thinking, 'Am I going to live and if I do live, what is it going to be like?' However, at that point, my goal is simply to listen to them. I want to know what they are thinking about life and death. But, objectively I know that they may very well improve and return to a reasonable state of health."

Jack then asks Susan to imagine an alternative scenario where a woman has been on dialysis and fighting a disease for a long time. This woman has been going in and out of the hospital for years. Every time she leaves the hospital her life returns to reasonable.

Every time she goes into the hospital she comes out again. Then one day she has a medical event when life for her no longer returns to reasonable. This patient begins thinking to herself that dialysis is no longer worth it and she no longer wants to live. But her family members are thinking that even though she has been in the hospital ten times she always rebounds, so why would this time be any different? They assume that of course she wants to live. Jack says to Susan, "It is different now because it is ten years later and she is in her seventies."

Jack goes on to explain that many times the patient may know what he or she wants, but making the decision to withdraw from dialysis is very complex. Patients don't only think about their fatigue and pain, but they also consider their family's pain and wonder how a decision to continue or discontinue dialysis will impact their families. Frequently they are torn between not wanting to be a burden to the family and not wanting to let the family down. According to Jack the most difficult situations are when there is a lack of unanimity. Sometimes in these cases the family has never discussed the patient's wishes, or if they have, the discussion has been forgotten or they aren't coping well with the patient's desire to discontinue. Jack reflects, "Those are the most uncomfortable situations, because you can see your patients struggle. They are suffering because they are unhappy with *how* they are living; they don't want to continue, but they feel trapped."

Jack then points out a very visible example of someone who chose to discontinue dialysis—the American author James A. Michener who died in 1997. Michener had been on dialysis for years before he made the conscious decision to discontinue. At that time he was ninety, his wife had died of a stroke two years earlier, he was reading, he was writing, his mind was in decent shape, but his body was failing him. In Jack's estimation, Michener, while it may not have been his intent, successfully raised awareness around the consciousness of choice.

Is it more likely for folks to want to discontinue dialysis when they are contending with other medical issues, in addition to dialysis?

"Sure, because the burden upon them is greater. It is a very different long-term view for someone who is young and can get a transplant than for someone who is elderly and has bad heart disease or diabetes and is not a candidate for a transplant. As time marches on it doesn't get easier."

Have you ever contemplated what it would be like to live on dialysis?

"Yes I have, and at this point in life I would do it. At a later point in life I might not. I once came upon a patient who was desperately ill with an infected gallbladder. He was in his seventies but you could tell he was very active. His legs, arms, and face were tanned. Clearly he was out in the world doing stuff. In response to the possibility of needing dialysis he said, 'No, I'm not going to do it.' Later I saw him at the clinic. He was on dialysis. He told me, 'Now I actually feel pretty good and I'm doing things that I enjoy. I'm going to stick with dialysis.' He had a change of mind, a change of heart, and a change of circumstances. His health improved and he realized that he actually was still alive. My point is you just don't know what you will do until you are in those shoes. Like I said, you go to the cliff alone. You walk there. You stand there. You feel the cool breeze. You see the depth of your decision. You turn around and there is nobody there. You've got to make the decision yourself."

Who's Who on the K-Team

Jack's story shows that nephrologists are somewhat unique in the field of modern-day medicine. Typically they have longer and more intimate relationships with many of their patients than other types of physicians. As another nephrologist said, "We get to know our patients better than most other doctors do because we see them so frequently." Jack also raises the very complex issue of a patient's consent and desire for treatment versus the alternative, which would be to abstain from dialysis, enter hospice, and end one's life. One doctor we spoke to said, "I know there are nephrologists who would never discuss this subject with their patients. A dialysis patient might want to know his or her physician's philosophy on end-of-life issues." Not many other specialists—aside from oncologists, doctors specializing in cancer—are as frequently in the position of bearing witness or even assuring patients of their decisions to pursue or abstain from additional treatment. Jack's story shines a light on the importance of finding a doctor who will not only provide excellent medical attention and judgment throughout your illness, but who also will get to know you and your family very well and will respect your values and beliefs on this very complex subject.

Clearly, trust and understanding are the cornerstones of an excellent patient-doctor relationship. Given the depth and duration of the nephrologist and renal patient relationship, we encourage you to seek out a doctor whom you feel you can trust and who will hold your wishes and opinions in high esteem. Essentially the best possible doctor is one who knows much more than you do and can share his or her knowledge with you. Ideally you will find someone who is willing, at the very least, to listen to your opinion even if the physician respectfully disagrees. And should you ever wish to seek a second opinion, we hope you will find the kind of doctor who encourages you to do so. For those doctors, even if they believe resolutely in their recommendations, will consider your personal commitment to your course of care to be an important part of your health care treatment.

In addition to seeking a physician who has these very important intrinsic qualities, you will obviously need to find a nephrologist who can capably oversee the medical nitty-gritty involved in your ongoing care. In fact, some patients care only about their physician's expertise and have little concern for his or her bedside manner. As one old-timer with eighteen years of dialysis under her belt said,

"I think it is important to find a doctor who knows what he's doing. Just being nice isn't going to cut it with me. Anyone can be friendly. You don't even need to talk to me, you just need to know what you are doing." Ideally you'll be able to find a doctor who is both caring and capable, but like this patient you may need to prioritize the characteristics that are important to you. Now, let's quickly review the important tasks nephrologists perform as well as the roles that each of the key members on your K-Team plays.

The Nephrologist

Your nephrologist will meet with you and your family to answer questions about your kidney function, dialysis, and treatment. He or she will decide how many times weekly and for what length of time you must dialyze based on your laboratory results and physical exams. Your doctor will also prescribe the needed medications to accompany your dialysis treatment. Your nephrologist will provide advice and guidance regarding transplantation and the various dialysis modalities. The nephrologist will recognize problems arising from acute illness or secondary conditions, treat them if possible, or refer the patient to primary care physicians or known consultants. Your doctor will work closely with your transplant surgeon and transplant team to prepare you for possible transplantation. And if ever the time comes, your doctor will be a resource, along with mental health professionals and clergy, to answer questions you may have about the decision to terminate dialysis.

The Nurse

Medicare mandates that a licensed health professional be on duty at all times while patients are dialyzing at a clinic. Therefore a doctor, a nurse, or a nurse practitioner must always be present. Most often a nurse will be the one to meet this requirement. Nurses wear several hats. They may conduct new patient, family, and staff training. They may actually put patients on the machines, monitor them, and take them off, or they may supervise the on-duty technicians while the technicians perform these tasks. Nurses may do rounds, meaning they visit with the dialyzing patients, and then report back to the doctor any questions or issues that arise. They may also conduct patient training of alternate modalities such as home hemodialysis or peritoneal dialysis.

The Social Worker

Medicare also mandates that the staff of every dialysis center include a social worker with a master's degree. Social workers are trained and qualified to assist patients and family members with the psychological issues that often surface once a patient has begun dialysis. Social workers can help address concerns about health, work, death, marriage, family, emotional or sexual intimacy, finances, and travel. They can provide opportunities for support as well as guide patients to resources that can help with finances, employment, medication costs, home health care services, medical equipment, or transportation. Social workers don't always have the answer to a question, but they are excellent at knowing who will. Social workers also assist patients who are planning to travel and will need dialysis while they are away from home. Once a patient's itinerary and destination is final, the social worker can contact dialysis centers in the area to make dialysis arrangements.

The Dietician

The dietician is a helpful resource when it comes to managing your new diet. On an ongoing basis dieticians will help you to read and understand your laboratory results so that you can continue to make changes and improvements. If you are not doing so well, they will offer suggestions and tips as to how to make better choices and replace foods that negatively impact your health. They can provide cookbooks and will often post recipes or weekly tips for all members of the clinic to enjoy. If needed, dieticians can also meet with family members to help educate them about your new diet and the ways in which they can be supportive. Last, when you are on track and doing well, your dietician will cheer you on. This person's job is to provide positive reinforcement and encouragement so that you will continue to keep up the good work.

The Technician

The technician is often the member of the team with whom you will interact the most. You probably won't just have one technician who always works with you. In reality, depending on the day, the technician who is taking care of you may change. However, typically when you arrive for dialysis one technician will work with you for your entire dialysis session. The technician will get you hooked up to the machine, will monitor your vital signs during the session, and will take you off the machine. He or she may be able to answer some basic questions about the treatment or the machine, but these individuals haven't received licensed medical training, so certain specific medical questions may have to be deferred to the doctor or the nurse.

The Patient—That's Right, YOU!

You are an influential member of the team and have the right to participate in decisions affecting your care. Yes, that is right. You hold power and you can assert this power in a few different ways. First, your ability to communicate effectively with your health care team will impact their ability to treat you effectively. The more concise you are in describing symptoms or issues, the easier it will be for them to determine how best to help you. Second, you have the power to ask questions, to disagree, to explain why you disagree, and to get a second or even a third opinion.

You may hear the words *advocate* or *advocacy* frequently associated with dialysis patients. Sometimes advocacy refers to a patient's involvement in influencing public policy and legislation. Other times it refers to a patient's ability to influence his or her care on a much more personal scale. In both cases the word advocacy is used because dialysis patients—or sometimes their family members—are, as we said, very influential members on the team. Jack even described the magnitude of a patient's decision making as "walking to the cliff alone." The number one premise of working with your K-team is this: you have the power to speak up for yourself and to be an advocate for your health. Once you embrace this philosophy you will be ten steps ahead of the game. The best quality of care you can receive will result from successful interactions among the nephrologist, the other members of the health care team, and you.

Other Members of the K-Team

Other members of your K-team may include the vascular surgeon who builds your access, the driver who takes you to and from dialysis, a physical or occupational therapist, the pharmacist, a transplant surgeon and the transplant team.

Unique Challenges for Renal Care Medical Professionals

Now that we've identified the roles of the team members, let's try to take a step back and look at the world through their eyes a bit. As we learned from Jack, nephrologists, unlike other types of doctors, often care for their patients for an indefinite and extended period of time. And with the longevity of care comes a level of intimacy and knowledge that many other types of doctors do not encounter. For some nephrologists this is a very attractive aspect of their profession; they truly enjoy this ongoing relationship with a patient and the patient's family members. For others, this can at times be a source of frustration as they never really "cure" their dialysis patients. They may have some patients who successfully receive transplants and leave dialysis, but they will still always be renal patients. For this reason, some nephrologists may miss the satisfaction of moving on to challenging, new cases. Essentially, nephrologists encounter some of the monotony that the dialysis patients themselves face.

This potential for feeling "burned out" is not unique to nephrologists. All the members of your K-team are susceptible to this sense of day-in and day-out monotony. We bring this up not to lay blame or deride those who work with dialysis patients. Our reason is just the opposite—so that we can recognize and sympathize with some of the particular challenges they face. As we said before, this is very much a team effort. As anyone who has worked on a team knows, the more we understand our teammates and where they are coming from, the better we are at influencing them and working with them toward a common goal. In this case your common goal is to keep you healthy and living well.

Getting the Most from Your K-Team

Chances are you will not see your nephrologist as frequently as you'd like. As we saw with Jack, usually the caseloads of these doctors are large, their responsibilities are numerous, and their time is in relatively short supply. The fact is, you may not see all of the members of your team—aside from the technicians—as often as you would like. Social workers sometimes do rounds weekly, doctors vary from weekly to monthly, dieticians typically round monthly. Nurses will often round and dispense the medications during your session, so you will see them more frequently. Depending on the team member's time constraints and beside manner, he or she may simply ask you how are you doing and then move on quickly to the next patient.

The bottom line is this: if you want to increase the quality and quantity of time spent with particular members of the team, you may need to make it happen. They may not be visible to you as much as you'd like, but you are on a two-way street and it is always within your rights as their patient or client to seek them out. Below is a step-by-step proactive approach that can be applied when working with any of the members on your team:

1. Start by scheduling a time and a place that is more conducive to having a conversation of substance. Respect their schedules. Rather than trying to speak to them on the fly in the hall, set a time in advance when you can sit down together and meet.

2. Give some thought to the amount of privacy you'd like to have during the conversation. If you want to be able to speak openly and in private then plan to meet when you are not dialyzing.

3. Write down a list of questions and bring it with you to your meeting. By coming to the meeting prepared you will be able to use everyone's time efficiently and effectively.

4. Try to be as specific as possible when describing physical or emotional problems, sensations, or reactions. Even keep a journal of when you are noticing particular symptoms. Jot down the date, time, and intensity or a brief description and bring the log in with you.

5. Bring a friend or family member with you who can keep track of the answers to your questions. Especially in the beginning, all of the information that you receive regarding your condition and care can be quite overwhelming and comprehensive. Because you will be trying to take so much in all at once, often it is difficult to retain and remember everything. Having another person, who can help you review the information even after you've returned home, can be extremely useful.

6. Ask for the team member to speak your language. By this we mean if your doctor, as an example, is using too many medical terms or is speaking in a way that you are having difficulty understanding, let him or her know. Don't be afraid to speak up and ask for clarifications or to just plain out say, "I don't understand."

7. This brings us to our next point: ask questions. Ever hear the phrase, "No question is too dumb?" Well, now that you are learning about the wide world of dialysis, remember this phrase

and live by it. If you have questions, ask. And if you have more questions, keep on asking. Be persistent. This is your life and your health. No question is too dumb!

8. Last, if you disagree with what you are hearing from any of the members of your team, feel free to respectfully voice your opinion and explain why you disagree. Also feel free to seek a second or third opinion when it comes to making substantial decisions that will impact your health and quality of life.

Being Your Own Best Advocate during Dialysis

We've mentioned already that you have a role on the team. Now it is time to explain just when and how you may need to step in to make sure you are getting the best possible care. As we said, the technicians are the folks you will interact with the most. Many of these technicians are extremely hardworking, good people who form caring bonds with their patients. Daniel has met and been cared for by many such people. On the other hand, technicians are not the best-paid workers, and at times this can result in lackluster hiring. We've heard from some technicians themselves that they have encountered sloppy colleagues who aren't always the most thorough or careful. To complicate matters, during dialysis the patient assumes the role of passenger while the technician sits at the wheel of the car. Or as one physician said, "The problem with some dialysis staff is they can very easily fall into the role of using dialysis and their power to push and command the patients. The patients are generally in a powerless situation unless they raise the roof."

So what do you do when you think an error is being made, but you don't want to offend the person who is going to be sticking a very large needle in your arm? Now perhaps you see the difficulty of the patient's situation. Once again we have some suggestions for how best to work with the technicians and nurses who will be administering your dialysis:

1. If you think that something is not being done correctly speak up and be persistent. Remember it is your life. As one patient said, "I remember a supervisor started to give me something and I told her, 'I'm not on that medicine anymore.' She looked at my chart and said, 'It says it right here.' and proceeded to continue to give it to me. Finally I had to say to her, 'I don't care what it says; you have to check.'" Admittedly the patient said this didn't go over well with the staff member, but he achieved his goal—he got the best possible care at that moment in time. Not only that, he said he'd do it again and he'd tell other patients they must do the same as well. Many of the patients we spoke with emphasized the importance of knowing what medications and dosages you should be receiving and keeping a watchful eye on the staff as they are administering them.

2. If you do have to be confrontational, try to do it as diplomatically and with as much charm as possible. Don't make it personal. Talk more about the issue at hand than about the person who is committing the error.

3. After a confrontational incident with a technician or nurse, kill them with kindness. For example, even if he or she was doing something incorrectly, as in the case of the supervisor above, thank the person for taking the time to check. Or, if he or she *wasn't* in the wrong, thank them even more profusely for taking the time to check. Don't apologize for your hypervigilance. It is your life. It is your right. But do thank them as graciously and sincerely as you can.

4. When you find that a technician or a nurse really brightens your day and is doing a great job, tell the person! Tell his or her supervisor. Give them compliments. Let them know. Everyone likes to be appreciated, and positive reinforcement is the best way to get folks to continue to do a good job.

5. Find out whether your clinic has a patient advocacy committee designed to raise issues collectively. The benefit of such a committee is that no one single patient is perceived as problematic. Donna, whom we heard from in Chapter 1, dialyzed at a clinic that was fairly progressive in implementing such a committee. Another dialysis patient who chaired the committee at that particular clinic told us, "We have a meeting once a month. We sit down and talk about any problems with the staff, machines, or patients. It is a good opportunity for communication. Or even just to clear the air. Changes have been made as a result. Some of the staff members and nurses have gotten better about wearing their gloves and washing their hands. And particular staff members have improved their attitudes in dealing with patients."

6. If all else fails, escalate your grievance to the head of the clinic or even beyond. Your clinic should have a policy regarding the formal complaint process. Often this includes filing a complaint with the state health department and/or the regional End Stage Renal Disease (ESRD) network. When registering a complaint, give clear and concise examples of the problem that you are raising. Rather than simply complaining about what is wrong with the situation, give concrete suggestions about how the situation could be improved.

Putting These Advocacy Lessons into Practice

Throughout the course of interviewing patients for this book we often heard them say that they have learned to speak up for themselves and accept a level of responsibility for their care. One patient told us that she was finding herself short of breath during dialysis sessions and she would finish her dialysis sessions with high blood pressure. Eventually she respectfully and calmly told the nurse that she needed to dialyze longer, and she wasn't planning on leaving the chair until her blood pressure was no longer elevated. She didn't lay blame or get upset. Instead she identified a problem and took it upon herself to make sure she received what she needed. As a result, the staff consulted with her nephrologist, and over several sessions removed nine additional pounds of liquid. Afterward, she felt worlds better.

What would have happened if this patient had not advocated for herself? She would have continued to feel bad, would have walked around with additional stress on her heart, and would have been at an increased risk for heart failure. Given the two options— possibly offending the staff versus possibly leaving her life at risk— it seems like a no-brainer to speak up. However, like this woman, many of us are shy. We don't like to rock the boat. Being assertive is not always a characteristic that comes naturally to us. If you are one such person you may have to consciously think about asserting yourself.

On the other hand, if you are very assertive to begin with, you may have to consciously think about how to be assertive without being aggressive. As one doctor said, "Sometimes people on dialysis become more impatient and more demanding. Especially since their life depends on the services of technicians, nurses, and doctors." The goal is to get what you need without antagonizing those who will continue to care for you in the future. Try to strike a balance between assertiveness and rudeness.

Important Resources

Part of knowing when and how to speak up on your behalf is knowing what resources and information are available to you. Two excellent resources for learning more about patient advocacy and working with medical professionals are these:

The National Kidney Foundation (NKF)
National Office:
30 East 33rd Street

New York, NY 10016
1-800-622-9010

To view an online copy of the patient bill of rights and a listing of local offices throughout the United States visit
www.kidney.org

American Association of Kidney Patients
3505 E. Frontage Road, Suite 315
Tampa, FL 33607
1-800-749-2257
www.aakp.org
info@aakp.org

Both of these organizations can provide useful literature and have members on staff who are well-versed in patient advocacy.

Last but Not Least, Thanking Your K-Team

Of course saying thank you is something that you should make a regular habit of. However, we recommend you find an opportunity once or twice a year to show a little extra gratitude for your K-team. As we said at the beginning of the chapter, they are hardworking individuals. If you've ever held a job in a service industry, you know that aside from receiving a raise, nothing quite compares to receiving praise from your customer. Providing the members of your K-team with tokens of your appreciation will serve two purposes. First, it will make them feel good about their work and what they do. Second, hopefully they will feel additional motivation to keep you around! How best can you show your gratitude? You can write them a sincere note of appreciation, make a gift, or even bake cookies. Your K-team will not be expecting anything from you. Arriving at dialysis with a gesture of appreciation will truly be a welcome surprise.

Over time, these men and women will come to know a great deal about you. They will see you at your best and at your worst, emotionally and physically. You and they will have good days and bad days. As you learn to trust and rely on your K-team for care, don't hesitate to trust your own instincts too, and speak up if you must. You may be the patient, but you aren't powerless. You have a say. You have a voice. You are an equal member of the team.

Six

Dealing with Emotions

The Psychological Impact of Dialysis

TRUE OR FALSE: people who are on dialysis are unhappier than people who are not on dialysis? If you answered true you'll probably be surprised to hear that a carefully designed research study has proven otherwise. The study, led by a psychologist, Jason Riis, while he was completing graduate work at the University of Michigan, compared forty-nine individuals on hemodialysis, three times weekly, with forty-nine healthy individuals of the same age, race, education, and sex.[1] All of the subjects were given electronic devices that prompted them to record their moods throughout the day. Moods were rated on a 5-point scale from "very pleasant" to "very unpleasant" and subjects were given the opportunity to answer these questions privately and repeatedly over time.

When the results of the two groups were compared, the researchers found that the levels of happiness were about the same for the two groups. The study also found that the dialysis patients overestimated how happy the healthy people would be and the healthy people underestimated how happy the dialysis patients would be. Why is it that we are so quick to assume that dialysis leads to unhappiness? On the contrary, we the authors have come to believe that if you were relatively happy before dialysis, in time, you will be happy after. Alternatively, if you were relatively unhappy before dialysis, you will still be unhappy after. How a person copes with dialysis and the attitude he or she adopts toward it is often reflective of how someone has managed to cope and the attitudes he or she has learned to adopt throughout life.

Of course, dialysis is initially shocking for everyone. This initial shock can cause a serious crisis for many individuals. Going on dialysis can result in depression, anger, anxiety, and even occasionally an emotional breakdown. It can also result in severe crisis in family relationships, which occasionally can result in separation and divorce. However, in these cases the marriage was suffering to begin with. Dialysis is simply the straw that breaks the camel's back. There is no question that individuals who have no other physical illnesses (such as diabetes, strokes, heart disease) often do better emotionally than individuals who have other major physical illnesses for the simple fact that their burden is lighter. But after the initial shock has passed and a person has become used to the new routines of the dialysis, he or she settles down to live life within the constraints of the treatment.

During this initial period of shock, what are the tools that a person can use to help ease this emotional distress? In this chapter we will identify and discuss some of the most common emotional responses to dialysis. In addition, we will recommend ways to help you deal with this emotional turbulence. The good news is that like most kinds of turbulence, eventually this too subsides. By addressing and tending to these emotional bumps, you may eventually, as the aforementioned study shows, find yourself just as happy as the next guy.

Throughout the years that Daniel has been visiting dialysis clinics we've met many rather well-adjusted, seemingly happy individuals, but most of these acquaintances rarely opened up to us about their trials and tribulations when first starting dialysis. Nor did they tell us much about the sources of strength they used to help them survive the tough times. But in the course of researching this book, Susan met Jeffrey, a pastor for a medium-sized interdenominational church who spoke candidly about the physical and emotional trauma of first starting dialysis and the important role that his faith played in helping him to cope.

Jeffrey's Story, a Hemodialysis Patient's Perspective

When Susan meets with Jeffrey, a middle-aged African American gentleman, he strikes her as just that—a gentle man. Jeffrey has been on dialysis for only sixteen months and he explains that he is still adapting to the transition. Like his father before him, Jeffrey suffers from diabetes that eventually led to his renal failure. His father, one of twelve children, had begun dialysis many years before. Jeffrey informs Susan that he also has six uncles who have gone on dialysis, and he says that he can identify at least four generations of diabetics in his family. Because of this genetic disposition Jeffrey surmises that he is the first, but likely not the last, of the second generation of family members to undergo dialysis.

Just four years earlier Jeffrey had been diagnosed with diabetes. And one year after that, he was referred to a nephrologist who told Jeffrey that his kidneys were operating at 40%. Jeffrey attempted to watch his sugar levels, but he didn't think he was headed toward renal failure or dialysis. Then two years later he noticed swelling in his legs and ankles. Every evening he would elevate his legs and every morning the swelling would be gone. What Jeffrey, who admits he was in denial, didn't realize was that the fluid was simply moving around from one place to another. This routine continued until one morning, as he was walking into the building where he worked, Jeffrey collapsed. Paramedics rushed him to the hospital and the next thing he knew he was being dialyzed.

At first, Jeffrey says he really didn't think about what it meant to be on dialysis. He just wanted the doctors and nurses to do whatever it took to make him feel better. But he soon realized, he did not like the catheter or the cramps he suffered as fluid was removed from his lungs and body. All told, during his week-long hospital stay the medical professionals removed forty-five pounds of liquid. After that week, Jeffrey says he was a different person physically. It wasn't until he went to his local dialysis clinic for the first time after leaving the hospital that dialysis began to impact him emotionally.

How were you affected emotionally?

"Well, my father has been on dialysis for about eight years, so I had been around it. I had helped him deal with his emotional roller-coaster, but now I had to face dialysis myself. I think what bothered me the most was watching my family deal with my illness. My kids told me that I'd always been the strong one. I'd never been sick. I'd always visited other people in the hospital and comforted them. So for my children to see me flat on my back made them feel very helpless. Having them see me this way was difficult for me. When I was in the hospital, my daughter didn't even want to come to see me. She didn't want to deal with it. Just now she has started to write some poetry about her experience when I went on dialysis. Finally, she is learning to express herself more.

"I think dialysis was also traumatizing for my wife. We were getting ready to travel, to buy a new home and do a lot of things we'd dreamed of when the children were grown. I think she just had never imagined herself in that predicament in her life."

What was dialysis like for you when you first began?

"When I first started I had a lot of problems with my graft. Not just anybody could stick me, and that was upsetting too. I have a high pain tolerance, but it was frustrating when I would get a less experienced technician. Also the trial and error of trying to find my dry weight was the most difficult part. I didn't really know how much fluid I could have in between sessions, how much would negatively impact me during and after my sessions. When I first began,

I was arriving ten to twelve pounds over my dry weight. That wasn't good. I would cramp during and after the session. Now when I come in, they take off two or three pounds. Unfortunately, I had to learn how to control my liquids the hard way. Until you start learning what fluid does to you and what certain foods do to you, you can feel pretty bad. Adjusting to a new diet was a whole other can of worms that I had to deal with. Over time I learned about my potassium, phosphorus, and calcium."

What advice would you give to someone who is new to dialysis?

"Really spend a lot of time talking. Talk about how you feel physically and emotionally. When I first went on dialysis I read some pamphlets, but honestly it was as if they were written in Chinese. They were filled with information. I think it would have been helpful for me to read more about the psychological aspects of what a person goes through in the beginning. I think visiting with a support group or seeing a counselor might have also been beneficial. I didn't do either of these things, although I did regularly read a newsletter that included personal testimonials. I found reading about other people's stories and what they went through to be extremely helpful. I also had my wife read the testimonials too. They were helpful for both of us.

"I would also recommend that new patients speak with the veterans in the clinic. Some of the folks here, the older folks (I'm the new kid on the block), they really helped me through a lot. They would ask me 'How are you feeling? What are you going through?' And they would tell me what questions I should be asking the medical staff. Having that kind of support and friendship was really very advantageous."

What advice would you give to a family member of someone new to dialysis?

"Talk to somebody about what you are going through emotionally. At first there are a lot of emotions that the family and especially the spouse are going through. But they don't want to share these emotions with you because they feel that you have enough to worry about. Despite this, family members also need an outlet or someone to talk to. I wish initially my wife had done that more. She held a lot of her emotions in for a long time. I think possibly talking to my father and mother, or somebody who had gone through the same thing, would have helped her a great deal."

Jeffrey says that when he first began dialysis his wife took time off from work to drive him dialysis. Because he didn't want her to feel like she had to spend so much time caring for him, he tried to get back on his feet as quickly as possible. Jeffrey tells Susan, "I think getting back to a relative state of normal where I could drive myself has helped a lot. I also think it helped that I opened up and said to her, 'Tell me how *you* feel.' I think she wanted to know what I was going through emotionally as well. This was important for her. It was difficult for me, at first, to share my feelings with her. In the beginning I didn't really like to talk about it. I would just say 'I'm feeling pretty good!' "

Interestingly enough, both Jeffrey and his wife were trying to protect one another from the distress that they individually were encountering. Jeffrey didn't want to burden his wife with having to take care of him. He didn't want to tell her truthfully how he was doing and felt that he had to rebound and adjust just as quickly as possible. Likewise, his wife felt angry and sad that their life was no longer what she had envisioned, but since she was the healthy one, she felt she couldn't share these emotions with her husband. During a stressful time the two tended to keep their feelings to themselves. Eventually when they began communicating more openly and honestly with each other they began to cope better emotionally.

In addition to addressing your emotions, what are some additional key success factors to living well on dialysis?

"Really, every individual is different. I think if it wasn't for my faith, perhaps I would have a very different outlook on dialysis and on life. Most of my life I've tried to encourage people to live well despite adversity. Suddenly I had to live as I've always preached. Along with my faith, I also have a strong support system in both my family and my community, which has helped me to stay positive and optimistic."

Are there any benefits to being on dialysis?

"Sure—I'm glad we have it! Dialysis is doing what my kidneys can't do. I also think it has made me a better pastor. I'm more passionate about habits that affect our lives in a negative way. I've only missed one Sunday at church since I've been on dialysis. The week I left the hospital I missed preaching, but the following week I was there. That first Sunday after I began dialysis I looked out at the congregation. I really looked at the people who had been sick. Many of the congregants had been ill for years. And I realized that our health issues are a collective problem. We live in a society that promotes unhealthy lifestyle habits. Now I'm much more conscious about healthy living and am an advocate of better health. I've even started a wellness program at the church for people to get their blood sugar checked regularly."

Jeffrey tells Susan he credits his faith, his motivation to help others, and the support of those around him as giving him the strength to cope, but he acknowledges that going on dialysis was tough. Physically it has been hard on him. Emotionally he has grappled with a sense of failure and weakness, fearful that he has let his family down. But fortunately Jeffrey's sense of accountability to his congregants whom he has preached to for so long has been his saving grace. As he tells Susan, "For many years I had talked the talk. Now I had to walk the walk."

Like the veterans he speaks of, Jeffrey strikes Susan as a man who has gone to battle with his physical and emotional demons and who has now crossed over to a safer place. In order to be a role model, Jeffrey was forced to find a way to cope. He admits his new schedule and lifestyle still require adjustments, but he also tells Susan he hopes to start traveling with his wife more, he is working full time, and he's looking forward to seeing his daughter graduate from high school soon. Susan can't help noticing that he is living well and enjoying life despite dialysis. Before they part ways, Susan finds herself contemplating what sources of strength or coping mechanisms she would draw upon if she were ever to walk in Jeffrey's shoes.

Once the Shock Subsides: Coping with Psychological Aftershocks

Like Jeffrey, most patients whom we met told us that it took some time for their physical health to improve significantly before they could begin to feel, much less deal, with the substantial emotions associated with this enormous life change. When they begin to feel better physically is when many patients start to feel anxious, depressed, or angry. Family members are also highly susceptible to these emotions. It is normal and understandable to experience them. But the people who do not do well on dialysis are the ones who cannot, over a normal course of time, address and move past these emotional states. Some individuals never cope well with dialysis. They think their life has been forever limited and they absolutely hate the thought of having to go to dialysis three times each week as long as they live—or until they receive a transplant. Emotionally, these are the people who do not do well. Now let's look at some of the most common emotions that can negatively impact dialysis patients and their families, what happens to those who do not cope well, and what coping mechanisms a person can rely on when working through these emotions.

Denial

Denial is often the very first reaction of many dialysis patients. Denial is a state of nonacceptance. When in denial, a person refuses to accept the fact that he or she is on dialysis. Obviously the person can see himself or herself receiving the treatment but chooses to believe that it is temporary and that all will return to normal in a few weeks or months. In this state a patient typically refuses to follow the diet or acknowledge the liquid restrictions. He or she continues to act and behave as before starting dialysis. The patient is neither angry nor depressed; he or she simply refuses to believe that life on dialysis is now a reality. As we all know, innocence can be bliss, but dialysis patients cannot stay in this state forever. It is only a matter of time before their denial causes their health to decline precipitously.

Sadly, many of the individuals whom we interviewed claimed not to have believed what the doctors told them regarding their diet and liquid restrictions. Too many said they had to learn to take care of themselves and heed their doctor's advice the hard way. This was unfortunate, because this learning path usually meant jeopardizing their lives. Denial, while common, is not a particularly helpful response to the newness of dialysis. As one physician we interviewed said, "Like so many things in life, dialysis is a head game. Most patients won't do well if they struggle and fight against dialysis rather than work with it. Denial or the inability to come to terms with dialysis prevents some people from doing as well as they might. Can you get by when you are messy and inattentive and don't comply with instructions? Yes you can, but if you want to do better you need to have your thoughts together and understand what is being asked of you. And by understand I generally mean you have to do what you are told." Patients are much better served the sooner they can accept their reality and work within the guidelines that are set forth by their medical team. One way or another, reality will eventually sink in and when it does patients are then most often confronted with feelings of anxiety, depression, or anger.

Anxiety

Anxiety makes one feel uneasy, fearful, nervous, and worried. Physically one can experience a quickened pulse, lethargy, irritability, and

increased sweating. There are numerous sources of anxiety that patients associate with dialysis. Let's start with the whopper, the big
kahuna of them all: anxiety about death. One patient we spoke with
had the very terrifying and unfortunate experience of watching as a
woman who was sitting across from him at dialysis went into cardiac
arrest. Sadly, he witnessed her death. And of course, one of the first
thoughts to cross his mind was, "That could be me. I could die."
And that was an extremely frightening thought. It shook him to his
core. His experience that day was extreme and unusual, but even
without having such a jarring experience you too may be growing
anxious over the thought that dialysis has brought you a bit closer to
your mortality. Before dialysis, you might have thought you were in-
vincible (although in reality you weren't) and now you know you are
not. "True, now that you are on dialysis, statistically speaking, your
chances of dying are greater than they were before your kidneys
failed and you needed dialysis." There we have said it: you may die.
Dwelling on this fact can be paralyzing and unhealthy. Now it is
time to move on. The good news about facing your mortality is that
once you realize you won't be on this earth forever you may actually
appreciate certain aspects of life more than you ever did before dialysis. However, becoming accustomed to this new level of awareness
can and does often heighten levels of anxiety.

Dialysis patients are often anxious about death, but this is not the
only common cause of anxiety. Many times they are anxious about
the actual dialysis process itself; they are afraid of the needles, of seeing their blood outside their body, of feeling pain, of sitting among
other patients who are significantly sicker than they, wondering if
the treatment actually will work as intended. Feeling acutely anxious
about all of the above is normal—for a time—but human beings
are remarkably adaptable. As the novelty of dialysis wears off, you
should become increasingly comfortable with what goes on inside
the clinic and the patients who frequent the clinic. No one wants to
get used to dialysis, but many people do. Or at least they do enough

to muddle through while taking ample pleasures from life. However, if feelings of anxiety persist indefinitely, it may be time for you to seek out additional sources of assistance. We'll discuss these resources shortly.

Now that you are dependent on dialysis to live, you may also become anxious about what would happen to you in the event of a natural or terror disaster. Of course, it is not likely that you'll ever have to deal with either of these happenings, but even so, this is not an unreasonable fear to have. In times of crisis basic needs must be met. For most people, their basic needs are food, water, shelter, clothing, and medical care. For someone on dialysis, being able to access electricity or supplies for peritoneal or home hemodialysis or a hemodialysis center is another basic need that must be met. As you listen to the world news and hear of the latest natural disaster it is normal to think, "What would happen if the power were to go out, the roads were to be washed out, or I was to be snowed in? What would happen to me, if I *could not* get to the clinic or perform my own dialysis? How long could I survive without dialysis?" These thoughts are scary, and while we can find comfort by being prepared for emergencies (see Chapter 10 regarding travel and emergency preparations), we can still get worked up and nervous by constantly imagining doomsday scenarios.

These types of "what if" questions bring us to another common source of anxiety: a fear of losing control. Many of us like to have a sense of control over our lives, days, actions. We think that by making lists, schedules, plans, routines, or goals we can influence the course of our lives. This may be so, but there are also events we cannot control that impact us profoundly. Going on dialysis is one such event. Losing this real or perceived sense of control is often the primary anxiety trigger for many individuals. For people who demand control, the best course of action is to gain knowledge and understanding and in some cases even pursue a modality that allows for greater self-management and care.

Last, many individuals experience worry and anxiety about how and if they will be able to continue to work and be a provider for their family. Financial concerns are a huge source of anxiety for many dialysis patients. Or, as we saw with Jeffrey, some people may be anxious about how dialysis will affect their family not just financially but emotionally as well. This sense of concern and responsibility for the well-being of their loved ones can be an additional source of anxiety.

Depression

By far the most common reaction to undergoing dialysis is depression. Statistics show that up to 40% of people with nonfunctioning kidneys experience depression at some point in time.[2] Larry whom we met in the previous chapter told us, "I wish I'd known before I went on dialysis that the toxins that were gradually increasing in my system as my kidney function declined commonly can cause depression. In addition to being somewhat more forgetful for the few years prior to dialysis, I know that I found myself emotionally overwrought at times. I certainly considered going into therapy and getting medication. I think it affected my relationships with my wife and children. I wish I'd known the emotional impact that the toxins were having on me because after those first three weeks of dialysis all of a sudden it was *sunshine*." In Larry's case his depression was corrected by going on dialysis; however, some individuals actually find the situational stress of dialysis to perpetuate depression. Or as Elena of Chapter 3 told us, "The first thing that will happen when a person begins dialysis is he or she is going to be depressed. You start treatment and you are *so* depressed." And to second that thought, a dialysis social worker whom we met explained, "I stop by every treatment at the beginning so I can see how the person is adjusting. Adapting to dialysis is not easy. Everyone has a hard time and depression is really common."

Symptoms of depression include feelings of sadness, loss of appetite, insomnia, difficulty concentrating, lack of interest in life, a tendency to withdraw from others, and an unwillingness to engage in activities that once brought pleasure. Patients often become hopeless and encounter feelings of despair when they learn that they have to undergo dialysis. Sometimes they see no light at the end of the road and some patients even become profoundly depressed. If the depression lingers, it can become more severe and can pose a threat to the patient's life. In the extreme reaction, patients become suicidal and occasionally attempt or even commit suicide. This is, however, very rare.

Depressed individuals often blame others (nephrologists, nurses, technicians) for their illness and refuse to take any responsibility themselves. Any problems that occur in the clinic are somebody else's fault. If the technician has a hard time sticking the needle into the access, he is incompetent. If the patient becomes light-headed or nauseous, it is the nurse's fault. It is always somebody else's problem. The fact that a person has a serious illness and that the machine literally saves his or her life is not something that the individual can appreciate in this state.

Like anxiety, depression can be short-lived and pass after a number of days. However, if depression persists longer than a few weeks, once again there are resources available to help you move on. It is important that you communicate openly and honestly with your doctor and social worker about how you are feeling emotionally. If you do so, they will be able to identify when you might need counseling or medication to help treat your depression. Sometimes when we are depressed, we are the last ones capable of identifying or diagnosing our depression.

Anger

Feelings of depression and despair can easily mutate into anger. When patients feel tremendously sorry for themselves, they at times become enraged at themselves, their loved ones, the caretakers, anyone within earshot. They are so furious that they have been given a raw deal in life that they scream, yell, curse, and at the end of the day, do not feel better. Of course, wondering "Why me?" is normal for a while. Yet if the patient cannot move past this sense of injustice, a constant lament of "Woe is me" can become toxic and antiproductive. These patients have temporarily lost an important part of living with adversity. They can no longer take a step away from themselves and realize that they should be grateful to be alive. Yes, they have to go to a clinic three times a week as long as they live or until they receive a transplant. And yes, even if they travel to the end of the earth, they still have to be on dialysis three times a week. But they can work, play, make love, and enjoy most of their waking hours each week. However, an ongoing sense of anger and frustration at the world prevents them from seeing this reality. Like anxiety and depression, anger is a completely understandable emotion for an individual to experience when first starting dialysis. However, learning to release this anger and move on is necessary in order to enjoy an improved quality of life.

One patient told us that when he began dialysis, his family suffered a great deal from the severity of his moods. He found that he was angry at them all the time. He told us that he wished he had understood how his transition to dialysis was impacting him emotionally. Had he known that anger was a normal response he might have tried to redirect it elsewhere, or, at least by acknowledging it, he might have been able to control it better. However, at the time he didn't understand that he was just so very angry about having to go on dialysis. He wasn't able to express or communicate his anger appropriately. He attempted to keep it bottled and hidden. However, his rage boiled up anyway and he found fault with everything and everyone around him. In time he learned to live with his lot, his anger subsided, and his home life improved. But he still regrets the way he treated his loved ones and wishes that he had been more self-aware as to what was happening with him emotionally.

Paranoia and Psychosis

Unlike anger, which is quite common among dialysis patients, paranoia and psychosis are two relatively uncommon emotional reactions, but still worth noting here. For a very small percentage of individuals, dialysis can lead to these highly troubled emotional states. We have witnessed a few individuals on dialysis who were extremely paranoid. In these cases and others, patients are not simply anxious or angry. They take their anger a step farther and believe that everyone, other than themselves, is responsible for their problems. They truly believe that all the people who care for them—the doctors, nurses, technicians—are determined to hurt them. Dialysis is a conspiracy to ruin their lives and they have been victimized by poor care. They may often yell or scream at the staff, sharing their deluded views with everyone in shouting distance.

Another response to dialysis is to have a complete mental breakdown or what the medical establishment would call a psychotic break. Dialysis doesn't cause the breakdown. Rather, a patient is significantly mentally ill to begin with, and dialysis simply pushes the individual over the edge. A patient who has a breakdown loses the ability to think rationally, often acts out violently, may attempt to pull out needles during a dialysis session, and may require restraints in order to sit still throughout a treatment. This is not a pleasant scene for other patients to witness. Given its rarity, we simply raise this reaction to dialysis in hopes of preparing you, should you be in the uncomfortable position of witnessing such a disturbance. In instances of patients suffering from mental illnesses of great magnitude, either paranoia or psychosis, psychiatric treatment including medication can be initiated and patients can improve markedly.

Healthy Coping Mechanisms and Resources

What if you cannot get past your normal feelings of anxiety or depression or anger? What then? Well, you may need some assistance. Assistance comes in many shapes and sizes and there is no shame in needing help emotionally. As we've heard before, starting dialysis is a big deal. Usually events of this magnitude present emotional hurdles that must be overcome. You may think that you are doing fine, but if you can't sleep at night, or if you are breaking into a cold sweat every time your dialysis machine beeps, or if you notice that everyone from the receptionist to the technician seems to be giving you dirty looks in response to your behavior, then it might be time to acknowledge that you aren't coping so well. There are several resources available to you. Usually the hardest step is knowing to ask for help and knowing that this is not a sign of weakness. In actuality it is just the opposite; it is a sign of strength to be able to know when you need support. The most common sources of assistance in coping include family and friends, professional counselors, support groups, medication, faith, and spirituality.

Family and Friends

As we saw with Jeffrey, his first reaction toward dialysis was to try to be strong for his family. He didn't want them to worry and so he didn't really let them in or tell them what he was going through. The people with whom he felt the most comfortable sharing his concerns and feelings turned out to be his new friends, the other patients whom he met at his clinic. He found that talking with them was an excellent source of comfort and information. And in time he did begin to open up to his spouse, which he admits really helped both of them emotionally. There is a difference between complaining and communicating. Being able to introduce your loved ones to what you are experiencing is an important step in the coping process. In the past, Daniel has commented to Susan that having Margie in his life "makes dialysis significantly more bearable." He added, "I feel that I have an ally, someone who could go through the battles with me, which makes a huge difference." We hope that all our readers are fortunate enough to have someone like that in their lives.

Other family members—for example, young children or adolescents living at home—occasionally find it difficult to deal with the dialysis patient. The illness should be carefully explained to them, and as much as possible, they too should be part of the team.

A fine balance needs to be struck between support and reliance. Leaning on your loved ones for concern and understanding is important. Yet both the family members and the patients themselves should be careful not to underestimate the patient's capabilities. In other words, dialysis patients shouldn't be babied too much or too long. It is important for dialysis patients to reclaim their independence and productivity as much as possible.

Despite this, the spouse of the dialysis patient often does have to spend some of her or his time taking care of the dialysis patient. Even under the best circumstances, three times a week the patient comes home from dialysis and he or she is weak, tired, and in need of a little extra attention. The four non-dialysis days are usually better, and the patient can take care of himself or herself. As the weeks roll into months and years, the caregiver needs to have what has been called "respite care." The spouse of the dialysis patient needs to do something for himself or herself that does not involve the patient. For example, a spouse can go to a resort, go hiking, visit relatives in another city or country, or even just go to a movie or a theater performance. On returning, he or she will feel reenergized.

Margie is a huge advocate of the benefits of respite care. Over the years, off and on she's experienced periods of feeling burned out. Not often, but at times, she experiences a weariness that comes with increased worrying about Daniel's health. Since Daniel went on dialysis,

Margie has been fortunate enough to take an annual trip on her own. Most notably, she has gone hiking and camping with tour groups in National Parks throughout the United States and Canada. Daniel is not a fan of camping or hiking, which is why these trips are a particularly good outlet for Margie. Although he misses her, he is not resentful of her experience and she is able to do something she loves, something that is just for her. Her weeks outdoors are very rejuvenating and she returns home ready to resume her routine of providing tender loving care and encouragement for Daniel.

Professional Counselors

Although we often want to rely on friends and family members to provide all the help we'll need, sometimes when they are also trying to cope they can't always provide the most objective or adequate counsel. Especially in the beginning, as we've mentioned, family members are often struggling themselves with the new circumstances. To have an open line of communication is important, but it is equally important to realize a family member or friend's limitations. Sometimes we may benefit from the expertise of an unbiased professional who is trained to help individuals undergoing stress and emotional upheaval. Every dialysis clinic has a social worker on staff. Social workers wear many hats including that of travel expert and financial counselor. However, their intended role is to provide psychological counseling and emotional support to dialysis patients and their families. Although many patients do not want to spend one minute longer than necessary at the dialysis clinic, they may be well served to make an appointment to talk with the social worker. Or, you can even ask the social worker to come and meet with you while you are dialyzing. Sometimes social workers may even refer a patient to a counselor outside the clinic. The costs of an external counselor may be partially or completely covered by Medicare.

Daniel is a psychiatrist by trade and has spent a lifetime treating individuals in need of emotional assistance. When he first went on dialysis he himself sought out the help of a psychiatrist outside of his clinic with whom he could meet weekly. Margie did as well. They found having someone to talk with confidentially who could be completely objective and willing to listen to what they were going through was helpful. Similar resources are available to you if you seek them out.

Support Groups

The social worker at the clinic will also be knowledgeable of any support groups in the area for dialysis patients and their families. Many times just hearing that what you are going through is normal and that others are experiencing the exact same thing can be a great source of comfort. There are also support groups for individuals awaiting transplants, and you may be interested in investigating one of these. Like the community in the dialysis center, support groups can assume healthy or unhealthy dynamics. When you attend a support group, it is important to try to gauge which type of group you have found. Is it the type that truly provides support, helpful tips, and inspirational stories? Or is the type that quickly dissolves into a black hole of complaining, negativity, and wallowing? If you've arrived at the first kind, great! This might be a good place for you to help process all the changes going on in your life among other people who can really understand and relate. However, if you've landed with the second kind, leave and don't return! Attitudes can be contagious, and sticking with an unhealthy group dynamic can make you susceptible to catching these negative bugs.

Medications

Your nephrologist or your psychiatrist, if you are referred to one, can determine whether your anxiety or depression should be treated with the use of medications. If anxiety or depression becomes paralyzing, debilitating, persistent, and generally preventive of your ability to enjoy life, then medications may be in order. Many dialysis patients and family members benefit from the use of anti-anxiety and antidepressant medications. Fortunately, we live in a day and age when the types of medications available are very effective, and many have minimal side effects. There is no weakness in turning to medications for help, and there is no reason to be a martyr or suffer needlessly. There is no shame in using medications to care for your mental health just as you would use medications to care for your physical health.

Faith and Spirituality

Jeffrey spoke of his faith as grounding him and helping him to cope with his life on dialysis. A belief in God or a higher power can be comforting and reassuring to many during times of hardship. Spirituality can take on various different forms depending on one's beliefs. Being able to acknowledge that we are not in control and that there is someone or something far greater than us can be especially helpful in overcoming anxiety, depression, and anger.

Spirituality may include meditation, prayer, or attendance at a house of worship. Talking with a priest, cleric, or rabbi about life on dialysis and what you are dealing with can also be an excellent outlet. Spiritual leaders can often provide compassion, understanding, and advice. Typically, they have experience with helping members of their community cope with adversity; as a result, they may be able to share the collective wisdom they've gained by counseling others who have turned to them for solace.

Whether you opt to rely on family, friends, a support group, a social worker, psychologist, psychiatrist, your faith, spirituality, and/or medications, it is important to remember you need not take this journey alone. There are numerous resources available to help you weather the storm until you can reach calm waters.

Once the Storm Has Passed, Maintaining a Positive Outlook

Once you've dealt with the initial shock, anxiety, depression, and anger, you will still need to cope with dialysis one day at a time for as long as you are receiving this treatment. Over time, most people find that being happy while living on dialysis becomes progressively easier. However, you may have setbacks along the way; when these arise you may need to rely a bit more heavily on the coping mechanisms we've outlined above. But when the worst has passed, what are the day-to-day techniques you can employ to ensure that you maintain a good outlook on life? There are several. Many listed below have earned their own chapter in this book, but we'd be remiss not to mention them briefly here as they are the most common techniques mentioned by dialysis patients and health care providers alike:

1. *Laughter.* As we read in Chapter 4, laughter is critical. Almost every person we met with said the ability to laugh and not take life so seriously was liberating and rejuvenating. And one patient told us, "If I didn't have humor I'd probably be dead right now."

2. *Work or volunteerism.* Finding a reason to be and to contribute to others can provide an ongoing wealth of self-esteem and self-confidence.

3. *Exercise.* Exercise has been proven effective at positively enhancing our moods through the chemical release of endorphins.

4. *Travel.* Travel breaks down the monotony of the dialysis schedule. It may not introduce spontaneity back into life, but it does transport a person to an entirely different place for a period of time.

5. *Knowledge.* Knowledge is power and it is why we decided to write this book. By learning about your disease and your treatment you can lessen your fears and concerns.

The more you are able to put these suggestions into action, the less you will have to work at staying positive: it should come naturally. As it does, if you watch, you may notice something interesting beginning to happen. Healthy people, whom you encounter during your daily walk of life, will not shy away. In fact, they will enjoy your company. They may not even realize you are on dialysis and might even be astonished to find out. Or if they do know you are on dialysis, they may even begin to admire and look up to you for your ability to live well in the face of adversity. You will become a role model. Of course, the main reward of coping well is being content with life. This is our primary wish for our readers. But the unexpected respect and admiration of others can be a very welcome secondary benefit.

Seven

The Impact of Dialysis on Interpersonal Relationships

Love, Sex, Family, and Friendship

Toss a rock into a body of water and watch as the water cascades from where the rock hits the surface. Now imagine that someone on dialysis is much like that rock being tossed into the water. The impact on the water is greatest at the center, the location of where the rock hits the surface. But, like the cascading water around the rock, those around a person on dialysis feel the reverberations of the impact and are profoundly affected as well. The more intimate you are with the person, the larger the ripple. Spouses, children, parents, and others very close to the person must endure the strongest impact. Those on the outer periphery—for example, a coworker or a simple acquaintance—may feel only the slightest blip or even calm. This chapter is written to help those near and dear to a dialysis patient ride the waves of dialysis successfully and to help patients understand the inevitable reverberations taking place around them.

This ripple effect was articulated by Keith, a middle-aged African American man whom a social worker had identified as someone living well on dialysis. In total, Keith had spent four plus years on dialysis—three and a half on hemodialysis and one on peritoneal.

Although Keith performed peritoneal dialysis from the comfort of his home, he and Susan agreed to meet in an empty room at the dialysis center where he'd periodically go to have his labs tested. As he signed the consent form that assured him of anonymity, Keith said, "Go ahead and use my name if you want. Whatever I tell you, I'd tell anyone. I'm an open book." Despite his assurances, we felt compelled to mask his true identity.

Keith's Story, a Perspective of a Peritoneal Dialysis Patient

During the course of their conversation Susan learned that Keith had not had the easiest life. Both he and his wife were recovering drug addicts and alcoholics. At the time of the interview, he had been sober for eleven years and his wife for ten. His kidney failure was discovered during an optional routine blood check provided by his employer. His tests showed that he was perilously close to needing dialysis. Feeling perfectly fine at the time, Keith was stunned. In fact, he didn't believe the doctors and refused to have an access built until his body became so bloated with fluids that the physicians explained he would die without immediate treatment.

Keith told Susan the doctors were unable to declare with certainty the cause for his kidney decline, but off and on he has wondered if it was from the years of drug and alcohol abuse. Now he simply chalks it up to fate. During the course of the interview Keith opened up to Susan about some of the most sensitive and intimate details of his family, marital, and sexual life after having gone on dialysis.

Have you found that peritoneal dialysis is better than hemodialysis?

"I like it better as far as lifestyle goes. I can dialyze from home in the evenings. Also I hated the huge needles that they use for hemodialysis. I've seen some people's arms beaten up from years of injections and

I didn't want that. On the flip side, they put the catheter down so low in my abdomen that it can be aggravating when my pants aren't loose enough. You have to be conscious of it at all times."

Has the location of the catheter impeded your sex life?

"Well I was about to mention that, but didn't know if it was appropriate. Yes it has. Now when I'm undressed I'm very conscious that someone can see this tube hanging out of my stomach. You always have to keep it clean and now I'm worried that my or my wife's body fluids will get in there."

Has dialysis affected your sex life?

"Yes, my sex life after going on dialysis in general—not just peritoneal dialysis—has faded drastically. So much so that I had to talk to the doctor here. He even offered to talk to my wife. She thought it was her. I kept trying to tell her, 'Baby it's not you; it's the disease you know. It has nothing to do with you.' But, she wasn't buying that. My drive is not there. Basically it is nonexistent. Dialysis has been disastrous on my sex life."

Did you expect to encounter sexual side affects when you went on dialysis?

"When my kidneys first failed, everyone told me this was going to happen. But my ego kicked in and I went on a mission to prove them wrong. I went out and cheated on my wife. I don't know if that is an excuse or not, but that is what I did."

Keith explains that his infidelity created a serious rift in his marriage of sixteen years. After receiving a confrontational phone call from Keith's mistress, his wife left home for two weeks. Keith's attraction to the other woman was not singularly sexual. He described her as being "more someone that I could talk to than have sex with." Eventually Keith and his wife sought counseling, but his wife was extremely angry and upset. Luckily for Keith, his wife acknowledged that she had received second, third, and fourth chances during his first year of sobriety. At that point in their marriage she was still struggling to kick her habit, but Keith stuck with her. In return she decided she would forgive him this one betrayal.

What would you have liked to have read about soon after starting dialysis?

"I haven't read or seen anything about the sexual part of it. When my wife and I first started having problems I asked the doctor if he had any literature about sex and dialysis. He didn't. I think something should be available because it is a very real part of dialysis patients' lives. All the men I've spoken to have encountered the same issues. And my wife recently spoke to a woman on dialysis whose husband left her in part for the same reason. I think there are many husbands and wives walking around feeling like they aren't attractive any more."

How does your wife feel about your sex life?

"There used to be a time where I wanted sex all the time and she would push me away. I told her, 'I can't believe all these years I've been chasing after you and you've been pushing me away, and now that my kidneys fail you want sex every night!' "

How do you respond to her needs?

"I look at my wife and know that I need to take care of her sexually but it's just not there. There is about to come a time when I'm going to need to force myself just because and that will be awkward."

Are there other ways that your wife and family were impacted by dialysis?

"In the beginning I went from depressed to angry. I was pretty hard on my family when I first started. My ten-year-old daughter is the love of my life. She and my wife caught hell. I was grouchy. Mean. They weren't used to my behavior. Suddenly they found themselves getting snapped at for little things."

Do you think your wife was afraid you'd die?

"You'd have to ask her. She knew it was an alternative that I'd con-templated. At first, I told my wife that I didn't want to spend my life this way, that I just wanted to let it happen and die. She told me, 'You better suck it up and not cop out.'"

What role have your wife and daughter played in your transition to dialysis?

"Well my daughter was spoiled rotten and continues to be spoiled rotten! She and my wife are the reason I've managed to adjust. No matter how grumpy I get, they keep coming back for more. They are my support system and the most important part of living well on dialysis is having a support system. I can't stress how helpful they've been. It is just so important for people around a dialysis patient to be supportive through the good days and the bad days."

Keith's tale of infidelity may sound a bit extreme to some—and certainly is not representative of every dialysis newcomer's experience—but the inherent themes he raises—seismic shifts in his marriage, issues of virility, diminishing drive, care giving and support—are not uncommon among dialysis patients. What *is* uncommon is actually discussing them openly. Dialysis patients may talk discreetly among themselves, but from what we've seen and heard, very little information about interpersonal dynamics and challenges has been captured and made available to the dialysis community. In the rest of this chapter we'll discuss the different variables that impact those around a dialysis patient from the center of the ripple outward: from spouse to child to friend to acquaintance.

The First and Biggest Wave: The Primary Caregiver

Who Is a Caregiver?

Typically a caregiver is a spouse or parent, or occasionally an adult child who—aside from the person actually undergoing dialysis—will be impacted the greatest. For the sake of simplicity we will refer to the primary caregiver as the spouse, although we acknowledge that there are many situations in which this is not the case. As we describe the role of the spouse and the effects that dialysis has on the spouse, most topics of discussion (with the exception of sexuality) are transferable to other individuals who may fill the role of primary caregiver. Whether or not you consider yourself a "caregiver" is debatable. A dialysis patient is not an invalid and does not require round-the-clock care. In fact, dialysis patients want to be treated like anyone else. But they do sometimes have bad days, feel weak or tired after dialysis, or encounter medical complications. During these times, they will look to someone to lean on for support and to ease their fear. The person closest to them will by default assume this responsibility and by doing so will on some level step into a caregiving role.

Also bear in mind, for some dialysis patients, there is no primary caregiver. The patient simply takes care of himself or herself. For example, earlier in the book we met Elena who lived with her parents when she first started dialysis and then later lived on her own as a single woman. Having a primary caregiver is not a prerequisite for a dialysis patient. However, if you are married and your spouse goes on dialysis you will to some extent suddenly find yourself in this new role. This next section is directed to all those on the front lines. You may not be sitting in the chair, but you are the one who must contend with the nutritional requirements, mood swings, and medical complications that affect your spouse. While it certainly isn't the same as being on dialysis, at times it may not seem fair that your life is changing significantly as well.

Stresses on the Ties That Bind

As we saw from Keith, transitioning to life on dialysis can put an enormous strain on a relationship or a marriage. Over time, marriages go through ups and downs. When a husband or wife begins dialysis, it is safe to say that the marriage may encounter a "down." We speak from experience when we say that the introduction to dialysis can initially be rough on a couple. And rough is something of an understatement. The transition to dialysis, which is a stressful time, can really test the strength of a relationship.

Why does this happen? With the introduction of dialysis you suddenly have two individuals who in their own ways are dealing with an assortment of emotions that include but are not limited to guilt, resentment, fear, anger, disbelief, frustration, self-pity, confusion, and worry. Each one in his or her own way is grieving the life that must now change to accommodate dialysis. Now imagine these two very anxious, stressed-out people living under the same roof. Chances are they will have short fuses and will be inclined to snap at one another. Similar to Keith's experience, couples may take out their anger and frustrations at the closest easiest targets—one another. They may find themselves being very unpleasant to one another and may even grow distant. Generally speaking, they may have a very difficult time living with each other, much less loving each other.

Like many marriages that encounter high-stress situations, some are unable to withstand the pressure associated with these reactions. We have known dialysis patients and their spouses who have separated or divorced. Divorce is a part of life and dialysis patients are not exempt. On the other hand, a social worker who had worked with dialysis families for over three decades said she felt that divorce rates were very low among dialysis patients and their spouses. She suspected the low rate of divorce was due to the enormous amount of guilt associated with leaving a person who is sick. We really don't know if the divorce rates are higher, lower, or the same among dialysis patients as compared to the rest of the population. What we do know is this: during periods of adjustment to dialysis, marriages are stressed, sometimes to their limit. Some marriages succeed. Others do not.

If you are going through a rough patch, don't despair entirely. Bear in mind that time and patience can be your most valued friends. Significant life changes take time to adapt to. These changes will put demands on your relationship to change. If the relationship is built on a solid foundation a couple will successfully adapt. However, a spouse needs to be patient and allow for these changes to take place over the course of days and months. On the flip side, if the relationship is healthy and strong, dialysis may eventually bring a couple closer together.

Because dialysis is a humbling experience for all involved, it can make individuals have a greater appreciation not just of their life but of the people in their lives. Typically when we appreciate a person more fully, we treat him or her with a greater love and respect. If you are lucky enough to persevere through the changes and challenges of adapting to dialysis you may be fortunate to come out with an even more loving relationship in the long run.

Once the initial introduction to life on dialysis has been worked through and a couple has gotten into their new groove, they still aren't home free. Intermittent stresses and strains may come and go throughout the marriage whenever a new medical issue, whether temporary or permanent, arises. We liken this process to walking on a balance beam. Before dialysis, you and your significant other are confidently walking across the beam in lockstep one following the other. Then along comes dialysis and bam! You are both knocked to the ground. Hopefully with luck and perseverance you find your way back up on that beam. Until one day, a new medical issue arises.

When this happens, depending on the severity of the issue, you may tumble to the mat again (and with that comes renewed fighting, distance, disharmony), or perhaps the two of you simply lose your footing, wobble a bit, then find your equilibrium and continue on. And so it goes. Continuously finding your way back up on that beam and learning how to maintain your balance is a critical skill you must now master.

Asking for Help and Education

Finding your own resources for support and increasing your own knowledge about dialysis will be critical when seeking this equilibrium. Now that the person closest to you is relying on dialysis to live, you may contemplate what would happen if he or she dies. You may have an overwhelming fear of being alone. You may struggle with how to be more independent and less reliant on your partner for self-definition. You may be extremely fearful of your partner's pain and suffering, now and in the future. You may even harbor feelings of resentment or anger at this person whom you love, for putting greater constraints on your lives together.

In light of what your loved one is going through, some of your feelings might seem petty, selfish, and hurtful. But they are normal. Obviously you may not want to share these fears or feelings with your husband or wife who is on dialysis. Your partner is already coping with all he or she can handle. But keeping these emotions repressed will be a disservice to your own well-being and eventually to your marriage. They will keep you from regaining a solid footing.

If you find yourself overwhelmed at the thought of being alone, having a difficult time, or feeling sorry for yourself, it is important to try to talk to somebody. As we said, you may not want to burden your husband or wife. Your children may already be coping with the mortality of their parent. It is better to seek out a professional, a spiritual adviser, or a close friend whom you've found helpful in your life. In either case you might not always be able to approach those in your innermost circle because they are being affected too. Rather, you must go outside the circle to someone who has a fresh perspective. You may find that having an outside resource enables you to air your worst fears and emotions.

Finding someone with whom you can share and work through these emotions is a healthy and helpful response for a spouse of a dialysis patient. And it will help you come to terms with your new role and the resulting changes in your marriage. But when you seek an outside resource, do so constructively with the help of someone who is not a threat to your marriage. In Keith's case, he not only sought out someone who could reaffirm his virility, but he also sought out a sounding board, someone he could confide in. Unfortunately his choice of confidante was destructive to his marriage. A better route would be to proactively find someone who has no other agenda than to be helpful to you. This would include but not be limited to helping you improve and strengthen your marriage in the face of dialysis.

Just as you may have to seek out help, you may also have to seek out education. Margie found that when Daniel first started dialysis she also had a great deal to learn about the treatment. She encouraged the medical professionals to view her and her husband as a team, keeping her in the loop. Over the years she has continuously learned more about dialysis. According to her, you can never reach a point where you know all there is to know. Education about dialysis evolves and is ongoing. And in the case of Margie, dialysis has become as much a part of her life, albeit in a very different way, as it is a part of Daniel's. How she plans her days, weeks, meals, and vacations has been altered to some extent by his dialysis. The more knowledge she gathers about his treatment and disease, the more confident she becomes in coping with her fears and feelings toward the changes that have affected her life.

Let's Talk about Sex

Dialysis is life changing and it also can affect one's sexual life. Keith didn't hold back when describing the difficulties he and his wife were facing with regard to sex. And as he surmised, they cannot be the only ones suffering from these problems. There are many other dialysis patients and their spouses who are challenged by one partner's sudden lowered interest and sex drive. With dialysis patients there are two possible causes for this decline in sex drive. One is physical. The other is psychological. Physically, dialysis and the buildup of fluids and toxins between sessions can be draining. A person may truly have less energy than he or she had before the kidney failure. This is especially true on the days that an individual undertakes dialysis. Certain medications for high blood pressure or diabetes may also diminish sexual drive. Aside from an overall diminished interest in sex, these physical burdens can sometimes cause erectile dysfunction (ED) in men, the inability to achieve an erection, or in women vaginal dryness, vaginal pain, and/or an inability to achieve orgasm. Additionally PD patients may feel encumbered by an abdomen filled with fluid, which can make sex uncomfortable and potentially result in medical complications. This is one physical obstacle that can be resolved relatively easily by draining fluid before engaging in sex and filling shortly thereafter.

Psychologically, a dialysis patient may be contending with the blues, which can diminish drive. One may feel less attractive as a person and more self-conscious about physical appearance and the location of the access. Like Keith, one may worry about how the access looks and if the access can be disturbed or harmed during sex. This increased self-consciousness can inhibit an individual's desire to be sexually active. Alternatively, a spouse may suddenly be afraid to touch or hurt a partner's access. A spouse may also suffer increased inhibitions by his or her sense that the dialysis patient is fragile and may "break." These psychological barriers are all common, real obstacles that couples may face.

That is the bad news. Now for the good news: You do not have to kiss your sex life good-bye. As a couple you can overcome these challenges. Neither a dialysis patient nor spouse need suffer in silence. There are a number of crucial and basic steps to remedying the situation:

• Open up and talk to each other. If you aren't in the habit of discussing your sexual satisfaction with one another this might be hard to do, but you have to find a way to have a nonaccusatory or defensive dialogue about your needs. If this is a truly uncomfortable topic of discussion for you, then you may need to seek help from a professional counselor who can help initiate the discussion. This is the critical step to finding mutual satisfaction in the bedroom. Shyness around the topic must be overcome.

- Once you've determined what each person needs, find a way to compromise and meet halfway. In many relationships, even those that aren't contending with a chronic illness, there is often a difference between sexual drives. The challenge is to try to find a compromise that both parties can live with. For example, if one person would be content to have sex several times a week while another would be content to have sex once a month, then the middle ground might be to have sex once a week.

- Redefine sex. The key is to think about when you first woke up to be a sexual being. You need to think about what makes you feel sexual. There are many ways to share intimacy with a partner other than actual intercourse, but you have to be creative. For example, alternative options may include kissing, cuddling, massage, mutual masturbation, or oral sex. To protect the access, different positions may need to be explored. A spouse should be able to articulate what might be appealing and satisfying while at the same time seeking options that won't be uncomfortable or overly demanding on his or her partner.

- Pursue medical options if need be. For men, ED, also known as impotence, can be resolved regardless of its cause, most of the time. To begin with, a comprehensive examination by a urologist can help uncover the root cause of the problem. Depending on his or her findings, a urologist may recommend one of several treatments that may include changing medications; couples counseling; oral medications including sildenafil (Viagra), vardenifil (Levitra), or tadalafil (Cialis); hormone replacement therapy by gel, patch, or injection intended to raise abnormally low hormone levels; injectable medications into the penis that create an erection, such as alprostadil, papaverine hydrochloride, or phentolomine; vacuum device therapy, which maintains an erection through the use of vacuum pressure and bands; or as a last resort, surgery and the use of a penile prosthesis. A urologist will likely start with the least invasive treatment first and recommend more aggressive treatments should the initial ones fail.

Now to focus on medical options for women, a urologist or, in some cases, a gynecologist can help a woman figure out what is causing the problem and how best to resolve it. The doctor may recommend treatments such as changes in medications, in routine, or in environment; couples counseling; over-the-counter lubricating jelly such as KY Jelly or Replens designed to diminish vaginal dryness and pain; kegel exercises to strengthen pelvic floor muscles; hormone replacement therapy via estrogen preparations; vibrating aids; EROS-CVD, a device that places a suction cup on the clitoris to increase arousal and lubrication; or vaginal dilation with a vibrator or tampon multiple times daily. Again, most doctors will recommend the least invasive treatment first.

One nephrologist told us that he's had several male patients inquire about medications for their sexual drive. But he said he has never had a female patient approach him about sexual problems or pharmaceutical options. Furthermore this physician told us that unless approached he never inquires about the health of his patients' sex lives. When it comes to sex, he leaves it up to the patient to approach him. Bottom line, if your husband or your wife truly is waylaid by a lack of libido, he or she may want to explore medical treatments. A patient should not be embarrassed or ashamed to broach this topic with a doctor. And, it is not uncommon for nephrologists to refer patients directly to urologists when dealing with these issues.

In time, you will find yourself much happier and more sexually satisfied for having addressed these issues rather than sweeping them under the bed. Your self-consciousness will diminish and you may even find that like many other PD or hemodialysis patients your catheter or access becomes barely noticeable during sex. Instead it becomes just another part of your body.

And Baby Makes Three

When discussing sex we'd be remiss simply to address it as a pleasurable part of life without acknowledging that it is also a means of procreation. If you are on dialysis or involved or married to someone on dialysis, you may be wondering whether you will be able to have children. Sometimes men on dialysis have a lower sperm count. If you are planning to start a family you may want to have yours checked. However, if you are a male on dialysis and you find that everything is in order anatomically speaking, there is no reason you could not impregnate a woman and be a wonderful, loving father. This is also true if you *don't* want kids—and everything is working in that department—so a word to the wise: take care! Your kidneys may have stopped working, but for many men they have little impact on the ability to parent. Yes, as a father on dialysis you might be a bear sometimes, tired others, and you'll have a rigorous schedule. But this describes most dads we know. Hopefully you'll have a lifetime to compensate for these shortcomings, and your child won't know any life that is different.

If you are a female on dialysis, bearing children may be a little trickier but don't despair and don't immediately count conception out. While you'd automatically be considered a high-risk pregnancy, if you are interested in having a child you should speak with your doctor, get several opinions, and weigh your options carefully. As is true with the decision to pursue a transplant, every woman is different based on her particular set of health factors. We don't want to provide false hope, but we have heard of several women who have successfully conceived and delivered healthy babies while on dialysis. We've even spoken to one, Leila, and marveled at her tenacity.

If you've ever been pregnant you know it isn't always a walk in the park, but pregnancy while on dialysis requires an entirely different level of commitment. Leila was somewhat of a celebrity in her dialysis clinic. Everyone had heard her story and knew what lengths she'd gone to in order to have a child. Before going on dialysis Leila already had one child. Soon after she began dialysis, she and her husband tried to have another. Unfortunately she had two miscarriages. The doctors informed her that she'd likely never have any more children and one physician even advised that she have her tubes tied as a preventive measure of protecting a new kidney, if and when she received a transplant. Leila chose not to follow this advice. As it turned out, she was fortunate enough to receive a transplant, but after a few years it failed.

Upon returning to dialysis her doctors told her that there was absolutely no way she could conceive as a result of having taken the immunosuppressant medications needed to protect her previous transplanted kidney. Hearing this news, Leila and her husband stopped using any type of contraception. Sure enough, to their great surprise she quickly became pregnant.

For the duration of her pregnancy Leila dialyzed at her clinic three hours a day, six days a week, taking a break only on Sundays. By ensuring that she dialyzed every day, the doctors hoped to avoid a toxic buildup in her bloodstream large enough to impact the fetus negatively. Leila did deliver the baby prematurely, but his lungs had developed sufficiently that he was able to breathe on his own. Eight years later she has a healthy, rambunctious boy who has her constantly on the go. When asked if it was worth it, she replied wholeheartedly without a doubt it was and she would do it again. And when asked if dialysis got in the way of her ability to be a good parent, she responded, "Not at all."

Helpful Ways to Be Supportive

Being able to make it through such a laborious pregnancy surely was a team effort on the part of Leila and her husband. Her husband likely sought out creative ways to show his love and support during those long weeks and months leading up to the delivery. Although most people on dialysis aren't in the process of creating another life, all people on dialysis are being stretched physically. Likewise, there are many small gestures that a spouse can do, throughout the duration of dialysis, to be supportive and helpful to their loved one. We share with you here a few of the loving gestures we've discovered over the years.

1. Learn about the dialysis diet and how to shop or even cook for the diet. Adapting recipes and finding creative ways to concoct food that your loved one will enjoy is one of the most loving acts of kindness that you can express.

2. Inquire about the dialysis clinic and the people there. Going to dialysis is like going to work. It is a whole world filled with characters and stories. Showing interest in where your loved one spends a great deal of his or her time is a nice way of expressing interest.

3. Give gifts that show you care. Go out and buy small drinking glasses and replace the massive cups you have in your kitchen cabinet. Find a pretty jar in which your spouse can keep phosphorous binders. In Margie's case she found two jars one marked with an X the other with an O. Other thoughtful gifts are a cozy washable blanket that the person can take to the clinic, a beautiful pill box for some of the medications, or an MP3 player for keeping the individual musically equipped while dialyzing.

4. Visit the person at dialysis. You certainly don't need to go every time or for entire sessions. But popping in on occasion, especially as a surprise, can be like a ray of sunshine.

5. If your loved one has reached a significant dialysis milestone acknowledge it and recognize the person's courage and perseverance. For example, to mark the five-year anniversary of Daniel's start of dialysis, Margie asked all of his siblings and children to write and send cards. She surprised him with the cards and a gift from the whole family—a paperweight inscribed with the phrase, "You are a star."

6. Determine whether there is a time when a little extra tender loving care can go a long way. For example, when Daniel returns from dialysis in the evenings Margie makes a concerted effort to be home and to have a good dinner waiting. This schedule isn't applicable to many dialysis patients but it illustrates how Margie tries to provide a little extra comfort when Daniel needs it most.

7. Try to give as much ownership of health and health care as possible to your spouse. As we've said earlier in the book, patients often do better when they feel some semblance of control over their care. For example, Margie used to put lidocaine on Daniel's access before every dialysis session. Then she realized that he was perfectly capable and should be doing it himself. Sometimes it is easy to take the caregiving too far. Don't enable your spouse to become more of a patient than necessary.

8. Feel free to express benign disinterest. By this we mean, you can listen to your partner complain about dialysis but do it passively, almost as if you are listening with one ear. The goal is to listen but not add fuel to their complaints. Your loved one may not realize it, but this is often the most emotionally helpful response.

9. If you need to travel on your own for business or pleasure, show you care from afar. Call after dialysis to see how the person is feeling. Perhaps leave a card or a gift under his or her pillow as a surprise. If you are in the habit of cooking for your spouse, make some dialysis-friendly meals in advance. Bring a gift back with you.

Taking Care of the Caregiver

Showing love and caring for your partner is important, but equally important is taking care of yourself and creating boundaries. We've already established that whether or not you consider yourself a conventional caregiver, you are one. And the extent of your caregiving responsibilities will vary depending on whether your spouse is contending with complications, additional diseases, aging, or other issues. It is important to realize that you are at a heightened risk to become burned out, tired, sick, or depressed yourself. To be able to care for your spouse, you simply cannot ignore your needs. As Margie says, "You are running a marathon, not a sprint. In order to make it to the finish line, you have to pace yourself." First, determine what you need to do to recharge your batteries while away from your spouse from time to time. Rejuvenating activities may include massages, walks, visits to a salon, going out with friends, going to the movies, exercising, taking a mini-solo vacation, or even a longer vacation if time permits. Whatever your pleasure, make sure to find the time and to do it without your spouse. You will be better off for it, better able to show support, and better able to put up with your husband or wife's "not so good days."

As Keith noted, on those bad days a caregiver often serves as a bit of a "punching bag." Sometimes the spouse of a dialysis patient, by virtue of proximity, is the recipient of some of the verbal blows, sulkiness, and crabbiness that a patient can't help feeling from time to time. This is not a lot of fun, especially when you feel like you've done nothing to deserve this ire. But if you are taking care of yourself you'll be less likely to let it bother you. The moods will pass, and remember what Margie says with a smile, "Go with the flow even in a sewer." Meaning that even during the cruddiest times of dialysis you just have to move with it rather than fight it. Or if that saying doesn't inspire you then her alternative mantra is "There is no defense against kindness." Even if your significant other is treating you poorly for no apparent reason (other than the fact that he or she is completely fed up with dialysis and you happen to be the only one within shouting distance), if you treat your spouse kindly, your kindness will be like a salve that soothes his or her anger. Eventually the person won't be able to help reciprocating. However, this ability to go with the flow and give kindness even where there is initially none in return hinges on your ability to constantly build and rebuild yourself back up again so that your defenses are strong.

The Second Wave: Those Who are One Step Removed

The majority of people within a patient's world are far more immune to the highs and lows of dialysis, and they will fall into the category of being one step removed. For example, this may include adult children, good friends, or siblings—just about anyone who is close to the patient but who does not live under the same roof. In reality the majority of people in this group generally show little interest at all in dialysis or a patient's life on dialysis. People live busy, stressful lives and often just ask how the patient is and go on to other topics. Some are afraid to ask about dialysis. If they do ask additional questions they are often misinformed or ignorant about the treatment. Sometimes their concerns or questions are tinged with an air of surprise that the patient is still alive and able to get around so well. While it may sound harsh, the truth is that most people in this group tend to be fairly clueless and rarely make an effort to educate themselves. Sometimes this may be frustrating to the patient or those on the front lines, but it is a reality of life. Perhaps, for those who know very little about kidney failure and who take the time to read this book, they will arrive at a new level of empathy and interest. If you find yourself within this group of individuals and, after reading, wish to be even more in tune with your friend or loved one's life, we have a few recommendations of gestures that would likely be very well received and much appreciated. If there were such a thing as "dialysis patient etiquette" it would go something like this:

1. First, go and visit your friend, sibling, parent, or other loved one at dialysis. Don't be scared or deterred by the tubes and needles.

Remember that many dialysis patients are able to walk out of the clinic and lead very good lives! A visit may be uncomfortable at first, but it will be very illuminating. More important, it will enhance the relationship between yourself and the dialysis patient. All three of Daniel's children and his two oldest grandchildren have, at different times, visited him at dialysis. While some were nervous at first, Daniel asserts that each visit was an eye-opening experience that enabled the visitor to gain a more realistic perspective, and as a result be more empathetic.

2. Before you visit, ask permission. Of course, there is a fine line between empathy and pity. Both Daniel and Margie acknowledge that they are proud and do not want to be pitied, or viewed as having or being less than anyone else. For this very reason, some people may be hesitant to allow a person other than a caregiver to see them dialyzing. As an example, we met one young woman who refused to allow her boyfriend of six months to visit her at the clinic. She didn't want him to picture her in that light. She wanted him to view her like he would view anyone else.

As an aside, we feel she was entitled to deny her boyfriend's request to visit until she felt the relationship was at an appropriate stage of intimacy and comfort. But we also believe that if and when she was to become confident enough in the strength of the relationship, allowing him to visit her while dialyzing would only enhance their bond. He would be able to learn about an important but not completely defining facet of her life. And as a result he would have a window into her vulnerability and courage. In theory, if her boyfriend was a "keeper," these insights would only draw him closer.

3. Don't just visit the patient once, never to return. For many patients, dialysis is a big part of their lives for many years. If that is the case, you may want to pop in now and again. At the very least visit once a year. A short visit requires minimal effort on

your part, but will likely leave a large impression on the person you are visiting. You don't need to stay for an entire treatment, but even a half an hour will mean a great deal to the patient and will be a considerate expression of your ongoing love and concern.

4. Occasionally ask the person on dialysis about his or her treatment. Asking patients about the clinic and the people there is a gesture of genuine interest in their life. After all, they do spend a lot of time there. Similarly, it is nice to ask dialysis patients from time to time how they feel or how a session went. While they don't want to be completely defined by dialysis, they don't want it to be ignored either. By asking, you are acknowledging a big part of their lives.

5. Request a complete, written list of dietary restrictions. When a person on dialysis comes to your home, make an effort to serve or have foods on hand that are good for him or her to eat. Try to steer clear of cooking unhealthy options, or at the very least provide an alternative. If you understand the diet, you will be in a position to be more supportive and less likely to inadvertently sabotage a person's attempts to comply with the diet.

6. Be understanding that dialysis trumps any other activity. If you want a dialysis patient to be present at a certain event, you must plan the affair around their dialysis schedule. Daniel and Margie have taught their kids that every day is special and no day is special; in other words, all activities and events must be planned around Daniel's schedule. If Daniel is vacationing with his family and has to dialyze on New Year's Eve, then the family can celebrate New Year's the day before. Eventually one becomes so accustomed to accommodating the ebb and flow of dialysis that one barely remembers life before dialysis.

7. Try to assist the caregiver if the need arises. During times of additional stress, if medical complications arise, check in on both

the patient and the caregiver. When the caregiver is taking a well-deserved break, help out by calling or visiting the dialysis patient more frequently.

8. Take the time to express appreciation and gratitude to the caregiver for all that he or she does to help the patient—someone who positively influences and impacts your life—keep on keeping on.

If you are among the circle of relatives and friends of a dialysis patient and are able to take these suggestions to heart, you will find yourself much more enlightened about and comfortable with dialysis and all that it involves. Most important, by pursuing these suggestions, you will make it abundantly clear to the person on dialysis that you care about what he or she is going through.

The Third Wave: Acquaintances and Strangers

Of course an improved understanding of dialysis can enhance an already cohesive bond between friends or family. But what about people that we aren't close to in the least? Do they really need to know that we or someone we love is on dialysis? Probably not. Every encounter depends on the context. If you are visiting the emergency room and are meeting a nurse for the first time, then, yes, please do tell him or her that you are on dialysis. But if you are introduced to someone at a barbecue, then there is no need to talk about your health. There are so many other interesting things to talk about, and if avoidable, it would be nice not to be referred to as "so and so . . . he's (or she's) on dialysis." This goes for caregivers too. You don't need to be known as "so and so . . . his wife (or her husband) is on dialysis." Stand out on your own merits and interests. In time, after someone has gotten to know you a bit better then you can let them know about dialysis, but first let them get to know the other aspects of your life.

As an example, we mentioned that Margie occasionally takes trips on her own. She started out by telling fellow vacationers about Daniel's dialysis and why she was vacationing alone, but her closest friend cautioned her against this. "For one," her friend said, "you need a complete break from the world of dialysis. And for two, there is no reason to go into it." Now Margie chooses carefully if and when she tells someone during the course of the trip. She only mentions it if she feels it is completely appropriate. When asked how people react she says, "Most frequently they are kind of fascinated and are surprised that I'm so relaxed about dialysis." Most people whom she confides in usually don't know much about dialysis. If they express further interest, she considers it an opportunity to teach them a little about renal failure and dialysis.

On the other hand, some people aren't nearly as receptive. Dialysis patients may threaten some individuals who are afraid of illness and these people will be more likely to shy away. Do not pursue them. You will only hurt yourself if you pursue them. Some people are just like that. You cannot change them nor should you try to. If you are tempted to, stop and ask yourself, "What do you get when you continuously hit your head against a wall?" A headache! Really it's not worth the effort. Margie and Daniel both say they have learned not to take these rebuffs to heart. They simply think of how blessed they are to have wonderful friends, and then they move on.

To return to our previous analogy of the rock splashing down into water, we've now addressed three of the waves that ripple from the center outward: the caregiver; those who are one step removed; and last, acquaintances and strangers. Regardless of which ring you fall into, or if you are the center of the commotion yourself, the suggestions in this chapter are intended to help you brave the wake of dialysis and the disturbance that it may cause to your relationships. Human beings are remarkably flexible, and like water settling around a rock, most relationships eventually adapt to the unwelcome imposition of dialysis.

Eight

Work and Financial Implications of Being on Dialysis

IN MOST SOCIAL situations when we meet a new person, one of the first questions we ask one another is "What do you do?" For most people what you do is considered to be a big part of who you are. When someone begins dialysis, one of the first concerns usually is "What do I do *now*?" And in keeping with the logic that what we do is such an integral part of our identity, it is a safe assumption that wondering "What do I *do* now?" is really just another way of wondering "Who will I *be* now?"

The thought of having to adopt a new identity, one that includes the response, "I do dialysis, or I do disability" isn't really a self-portrait that many of us would be comfortable with or take pride in. This sudden loss of an answer to what had previously been a very straightforward question can be very challenging. For many people new to dialysis the idea of who they were and where the future was going to take them has unexpectedly changed.

In addition to these weighty questions of identity come practical concerns about finances. Soon after "what do I do now," the questions of "how will I survive," or in the case of a breadwinner, "how will my family survive if I can't work," almost surely follow. Dialysis patients may wonder how they will pay the bills or if they will be able maintain the lifestyle that they've built based on their previous level of earnings. They may worry if they will be able to afford to send their kids to college, pay for the children's braces, or buy a home. Of course, all of these questions may invoke worry and anxiety. If they are racing through your brain, don't panic. As we mentioned at the beginning of the book, one of the biggest societal misperceptions surrounding dialysis is that a person on dialysis is no longer able to work or study. As one renal care social worker said, "I have known many people who assume that once they require dialysis they can no longer work. I often felt that it was my responsibility to challenge that assumption."

This particular social worker had been working with dialysis patients and transplants recipients for over two decades. During that time she had seen people who were battling kidney disease work in a variety of jobs and fields. She saw everyone from dishwashers, to landscapers, to construction laborers, to factory workers, to business professionals, to doctors who worked and dialyzed. She told us, "The more time you spend at home sitting in your house, the worse you feel. The more depressed you are, the less energy you have. This is the reason that the articles I've read over the years strongly support the idea that people who continue to live their lives as close as possible to life before dialysis do better. Unfortunately, there are certainly people who can't continue to work and I help them through that process. But when people start dialysis, I try to set up the expectation that they will work and if they can't *then* we'll figure it out. At least I want them to see that *somebody* expects them to work."

It may take time, to sort out the realities of what one can or cannot do while on dialysis, but in the interim our advice would be to try not to make any premature, large life changes immediately after starting dialysis. Take a month off if you have to, but plan on returning to work. For some people that may mean returning full-time; for others that may mean working part-time, volunteering, or being active in church or synagogue. Time will tell, but first allow the dialysis a grace period to take effect and allow yourself time to begin feeling better.

When first starting dialysis you may feel so sick and so debilitated that it may be very hard to imagine ever feeling well enough again to hold down a job. However, how you feel initially on dialysis is rarely representative of how you will feel in the long run. Or alternatively you may be quick to think, if my life will be shortened shouldn't I enjoy every last minute, and is work really how I want to spend my time? But, as we've said many people live decades on dialysis. You do not yet know what the future holds so don't be so quick to assume the worst. Give yourself the time to be able to separate the forest from the trees before prematurely starting disability paperwork.

This is not to say, that the task of working and juggling dialysis is easy. Many times it is not. In this chapter we will discuss a range of issues surrounding work and finances that arise when someone is on dialysis. We will discuss a host of topics such as the type of information you should and should not divulge during a job interview, as well as information about health insurance programs, protective federal laws for people with disabilities, financial assistance programs, and flexible work schedules. Our aim is to help you gain a much greater understanding of how to make work work for you.

Maria's Story, a Hemodialysis Patient's Perspective

One young lady whom Susan interviewed was successfully doing just that. Maria, a young twenty-year-old Hispanic woman was in the midst of dialyzing at 5:30 A.M. when she cheerfully greeted Susan from her chair. Susan, unaccustomed to such an early work schedule, nursed her extra-strength coffee, appropriately named "Fog Lifter," as she pulled up a stool and sat beside Maria and listened as her story unfolded. Maria spoke of how four years prior, as a sophomore in high school, she went into renal failure. Before being diagnosed, she complained of constantly being tired, which her mother simply attributed to, "typical teenage laziness." But when Maria began coughing, her mother grew concerned and took her to a local clinic. The paleness of Maria's skin, the bags under her eyes, and the whiteness of her fingernails were all telltale signs of anemia. To confirm his suspicions, the doctor drew blood and a few days later Maria's mother received a call asking her to bring her daughter to the hospital right away. Less than a month later, Maria began dialysis. Everything happened so fast, Maria said, "It really didn't sink in for a long time." As Maria talked about learning to cope with her illness, finishing high school while on dialysis, and deciding what to do next, Susan gleaned a little of the situational and motivational challenges associated with working—or in Maria's case, studying—while on dialysis.

When you first began dialysis how did you manage to continue school?

"I started dialysis my sophomore year. I managed to finish my first semester but then second semester and my junior year I was home schooled. My senior year I returned to the high school. That year, I would go to school and immediately after school I would come to dialysis. When I was home schooled I dialyzed in the morning and then in the afternoon I would have school."

Did you have an active social life through high school?

"I had my close friends, but when I attended school at home, it wasn't the same. When I was home schooled I didn't do much with my friends. When I returned I was more involved and I think I would have enjoyed a better social life if I'd stayed at the high school."

Why did you or your parents decide to home school?

"After dialysis I got tired and I just wanted to go to sleep. Initially I tried to have dialysis, skip first period, and then arrive at school for second period. But I found myself skipping several periods in the morning because I just wanted to go home and go to sleep. The schedule was messing with my grades so my mother thought it would be better for me. I didn't want to leave, but it was better."

Did you consider changing your dialysis schedule to the evenings?

"They didn't offer a late schedule at my clinic at that time. I would have had to switch clinics, which I didn't want to do."

Now that you have graduated what are you doing?

"I'm studying to be a pastry chef. I'm enrolled in a one-year program at the Culinary Academy. I wasn't sure initially if I wanted to do culinary or pastry, but I love decorating wedding cakes."

What is your current dialysis and school schedule?

"I dialyze from five A.M. to nine A.M. I return home to rest and then I go to school from five P.M. to ten P.M. The schedule works well for me."

What do you think differentiates people who do well on dialysis versus people who become stuck in a rut?

"I guess the main difference is whether you can just deal with it. The people who can say, 'Yeah I do dialysis but I do other stuff too,' they seem to do well. And just because you are on dialysis doesn't mean you have to stay put. We have to complete an externship for three months before we graduate. I'm thinking about doing mine in Paris."

Are there any benefits to being on dialysis?

"Yes. You can get financial assistance for school. There are places you can get grants. There are benefits that exist specifically for those who are disabled."

What has been the biggest challenge for you while on dialysis?

"I think what I mentioned before, learning to deal and adapt to the situation. At first when I went on dialysis I thought, 'Oh, I'm not going to be able to do what I want to do.' In fact, after I graduated from high school I should have started culinary school right away. But I didn't. I don't know why. I would just go home after dialysis and that was my day. I would do that every day and every day that was it. I didn't do anything. Eventually I just got tired and thought '*What am I doing?*' Life was just passing me by. An entire year went by and I thought, 'What am I doing here living at home with my mom?' So I enrolled in school because eventually I want to be living on my own and doing stuff with my life."

Maria went on to tell Susan about her boyfriend, going to the movies, spending time with her grandfather. She explained that she was awaiting a transplant but had been on the list for only a year. Aside from being on dialysis, Maria struck Susan as a very poised, normal, twenty-year-old woman who had managed to work around the scheduling difficulties and physical languor of dialysis. Maria was a perfect example of the countless numbers of dialysis patients who, despite the physical challenges of the treatment, manage to creatively carve out their professional path. Rather than letting her inertia settle in permanently, Maria discovered a vocation she thought would suit her talents, tapped into the financial resources that were available to her, and pursued her professional interests. Like any other twenty-year-old, Maria's future was filled with possibilities.

Practicalities of Working and Studying while on Dialysis

As we saw with Maria, her school life did shift dramatically after she began dialysis. At first she tried to continue going to school as she had normally done, with the exception of skipping first period. But because dialysis sapped her energy she was unable to show up to school on time and maintain her grades. Home schooling wasn't the ideal option, but it enabled her to continue her studies and get the rest she needed. If only her dialysis center had offered an afternoon shift, she would have been able to go to school in the morning and dialyze after.

Unfortunately dialysis centers don't often have the schedules that best mesh with an individual's work or class needs. And, as was the case with Maria, many people often must mold their work or school schedules around the schedule mandated by their dialysis center as opposed to the other way around. Or—in the case of peritoneal dialysis, which offers greater flexibility in terms of scheduling—a patient may need to carve out time and space during the workday to perform a manual exchange. Unlike many people starting dialysis, Maria had yet to join the workforce. But many folks who have to go on dialysis are already employed. What if they must suddenly make some changes to accommodate their dialysis schedule? What will their employer say? What will their employer do?

Know Your Rights

Individuals on dialysis are considered to be individuals with disabilities as protected by the Americans with Disabilities Act (ADA.) This means that you have certain rights that your employer must honor. As stated in the U.S. Department of Justice's *Guide to Disability Rights Laws*, this act "Requires employers with 15 employees or more to provide qualified individuals with disabilities an equal opportunity to benefit from the full range of equal-employment opportunities available to others. For example, it prohibits discrimination in recruitment, hiring, promotions, training, pay, social activities and other privileges of employment. It restricts questions that can be asked about an applicant's disability before a job offer is made, and it requires that employers make reasonable accommodation to the known physical or mental limitations of otherwise qualified individuals with disabilities, unless it results in undue hardship."[1] Before approaching your boss, at the very least you know legislation exists to protect you and others like you. You are entitled to make certain requests that will enable you to both work and dialyze. In general, you should feel more confident in your rights.

Many employers when approached about creative scheduling or

finding space for a peritoneal exchange in the middle of the day are willing to accommodate these requests. Occasionally though, an employer may not be so receptive. If need be, you, your social worker, or your physician may need to draft a letter referencing the ADA. As one social worker said, "I have used the ADA as a threat, although I've not had to get involved with recruiting lawyers to advocate for patients. Any time you reference federal law it does raise an employer's awareness."

We spoke with a patient who found himself in just such a situation. When he first started dialysis he was working for the city collecting recyclables. This patient's nephrologist felt that the job would be too strenuous for him and recommended he try to switch to an alternative position working within the same municipal department. So this gentleman approached his supervisor and asked for a "reasonable accommodation." The supervisor refused and suggested instead that the employee resign and go on disability. The gentleman confronted his supervisor saying that he thought he was being unfairly discriminated against. The supervisor retorted that he didn't really care what the employee thought. So, knowing his rights, this gentleman filed a complaint with his state's commission on human rights. Three days later he received a call from his employer offering him a position in the customer service department where he went on to work for several years. And as a result, the complaint was dismissed.

Unfortunately we've also been told that there are ways for employers to skirt the rules set forth by the ADA. Rather than refusing certain requests, some managers will accommodate them. But they will intentionally make the work environment hostile and unduly challenging until ultimately an employee feels that the only recourse is to resign and go on disability. We sincerely hope that you do not find yourself in an adversarial position with your manager or employer. However, if you feel that an employer is directly violating your rights as defined by the ADA, you should strongly consider pursuing legal recourse.

Know Your Rights as a Family Member

What if your spouse, parent, or child goes on dialysis and you must help take care of him or her? What are your rights then? The U.S. Department of Labor's synopsis of the Family and Medical Leave Act (FMLA) states that covered employers (essentially employers with fifty employees or more for twenty weeks out of the year or public employers with any number of employees) "must grant an eligible employee up to a total of 12 work weeks unpaid leave during any 12 month period for one or more of the following reasons,"[2] which include, "To care for an immediate family member (spouse, child, or parent) with a serious health condition."

Most people think of FMLA in terms of having an ill or dying relative and needing to take two months off. What many people do not realize is that, provided you are an eligible employee, you can also use FMLA intermittently. For example, if you have to take a family member to a doctor appointment once a week you can use the FMLA time for those weekly visits and protect your job while still caring for your family member. Your employer is not required to pay you for this time off and every employer is different in terms of how much of the twelve weeks they will provide as paid leave versus unpaid leave. But at the very least, you will know that your job is protected under the law.

To Tell or Not to Tell, That Is the Question

When Maria ultimately graduates from culinary school and begins interviewing for positions as pastry chef, what must she tell a prospective employer during the interview process? Does she need to explain that she is on dialysis? The only question that an employer may ask about your medical condition during the interviewing process is if there is anything about your health that prevents you from doing the job. As one social worker said, "I use the example of somebody who has a bad back and is interviewing to work on a loading dock for UPS. In that case the interviewee *must* disclose that information." She went on to explain that anything that does not prevent you from doing the job does not have to be disclosed until after an offer has been made. At that point, some jobs require a brief physical or a drug urine test. This would of course bring your renal failure to light. If you no longer make urine, ask your physician to provide a letter explaining your kidney failure and willingness to provide a blood or hair sample instead. Under the ADA a prospective employer should be receptive to this alternative suggestion.

But remember, early in the interviewing process you need not disclose anything. As a litmus test ask yourself, "Will leaving my job half an hour early to get to dialysis prevent me from doing the job and doing it well? As an alternative, could arriving at work earlier in the day, or working from home later at night still enable me to do the job and do it well?" If the answers to these respective questions are no and yes, then you need not say anything while interviewing.

Sometimes people will be interviewing for a position and will want to know up front if the employer will be willing to work around a hemodialysis schedule or to accommodate a peritoneal exchange. As we mentioned, in-center hemodialysis schedules are unfortunately not set up for the convenience of patients. In fact, most of the dialysis schedules interfere with regular work day hours. Usually a patient can't complete the earliest session (typically ending around nine A.M.) in time to arrive before the work day begins nor can a patient start the last session (typically beginning around four or five P.M.) after the official work day has ended.

While interviewing, a person on dialysis may hope that the employer will display a willingness to find a work-around to this schedule. Interviewees may also be uncomfortable withholding information that, while it won't prevent them from doing the job, may start them out on the wrong foot with their employer. Therefore they may feel compelled (even though by law it is *not* required) during the interview process to reveal that they must dialyze and may require flexible scheduling. But here is another way that employers can get around the ADA. Upon hearing about the dialysis before extending an offer, they may then choose not to hire the person on dialysis. If smart, they certainly won't say that they are choosing not to hire this person because of dialysis although in many cases that may be one of the reasons if not *the* reason. They will have another excuse. Bottom line: if you divulge that you are on dialysis early in the process you are taking a gamble on the integrity and open-mindedness of the employer, and in some cases, it may not pay off. So think very carefully about what you choose to share with a potential employer and when you choose to share it.

Flexible Work Schedules

Now let's say you have taken a job or are already working and now find yourself on dialysis. How might you be able to work around some of the scheduling hurdles of dialysis? First, if you are doing peritoneal dialysis, likely you will have some added flexibility as to when you must perform a manual exchange. This is one of the perks of peritoneal dialysis; it is not quite as rigid as having to be at a hemodialysis center at a specific time three times weekly. Like a newly nursing mother who returns to the workplace and must pump her breasts throughout the day in order to maintain her milk supply, you will require a quiet, clean, private place where you can perform an exchange. And like a new mom, you'll probably find your lunch hour cut short in exchange for time spent taking care of business—your business, that is. Again under the ADA your employer must make a good faith effort to find a place where you can perform an exchange. And most will. They may not always be happy to do so, but more often than not they will be accommodating. And if they aren't, remember you, your physician, or even an attorney (if it comes to that) may want to remind them of your rights.

If you are on in-center hemodialysis, you may need to be a little more creative with your time. Some patients will arrange with their employer to put in extra hours either at the beginning or end of the workday to compensate for a late arrival or early departure. Other patients may commit to working extra hours in the evenings or even while dialyzing by making themselves available via cell phone for work conversations and by working via a laptop computer at the center. As an example, teachers or professors will grade papers or work on lesson plans while dialyzing. One physician on dialysis returned all his patients' calls and completed his dictation, allowing him to have time to spend with his wife when the dialysis session was over. Other patients may work out a part-time agreement to put in a ten-hour workday Monday, Wednesday, and Friday. Then they take Tuesdays and Thursdays off so that they can dialyze on those days in addition to Saturday. We met with one gentleman who had been working at an insurance company for only six months when he suddenly became sick and had to go on dialysis. His manager allowed him to move to this three days a week part-time schedule despite his short tenure at the company. By switching to this schedule, the gentleman was able to keep his benefits while having time to dialyze on Tuesdays, Thursdays, and Saturdays. As one can imagine, he was eternally grateful to his employer for being so flexible.

If you are not sure how best to approach your employer or what type of plan might be well received, first meet with your social worker to strategize. Social workers will have seen many different employer/employee solutions and may be able to suggest a mutually beneficial proposal that you would not have thought of on your own.

Best Odds Companies

Now let's imagine a young woman on dialysis, such as Maria, but instead of attending culinary school she is pursuing a degree in business management. Once she has completed her degree, how can she determine which companies may have the best benefits and be the most accommodating in terms of her dialysis? As far as we know, a list of "Best companies to work for when dealing with a chronic illness" does not exist. However, the seasoned social worker we met earlier told us she typically encourages patients to look at larger companies. Why? First, small businesses typically can't afford the health insurance premiums associated with chronically ill employees whereas a large business with hundreds or even thousands of employees is generally impacted less by a handful of chronically ill employees. While their premiums do go up, they are better able to manage their overall costs due to economies of scale. For this same reason, they also tend to have better insurance packages. So not only would you be more likely to get hired by a large employer, but you would also be more likely to have better health care benefits.

As for finding an employer that will be receptive to a flexible schedule provided you get your work done, there are three lists you may want to reference: *Working Mother* magazine's 100 Best Companies, *Fortune* magazine's 100 Best Companies to work for in America, and the Fortune 500. While you may have no interest in maternity leave or on-site daycare, you can be assured that a company will not make it onto the Working Mother's list if it is opposed to flexible work arrangements. Hence, this is why you, a person potentially seeking flexibility, would also find interest in such a list. As for the Best Companies to Work for in America, each company may have a variety of reasons for making it onto the list and not all may pertain to your needs. But often *Fortune* will include brief explanations as to why a company has been chosen and again you can look for key words such as telecommuting, flexible schedules, job-sharing, and the like. If you cannot find companies on either of these lists that have operations in your home town or nearby, check out Fortune 500. Of course, just because a company is big doesn't mean that it is flexible. But the Fortune 500 lists the largest 500 companies in the United States and will help you to at least identify whether there are any very large employers in your area. Last, when seeking open-minded employers you may want to check with your town or city to find out whether there is an office of people with disabilities and if so, if they ever hold job fairs. If in fact they do, see if you can get a list of companies that have attended in the past. Odds are that those companies will be receptive and supportive of your dialysis requirements.

Standing Out from the Crowd versus Fitting In

Most of us want to differentiate ourselves in the workplace based on our work ethic, performance, and talents. In these cases, being seen as "different" from the rest is often a positive. However, being perceived as "different" because you are on dialysis is not a point of differentiation that many people are comfortable with. Like the rest of the population, co-workers can sometimes be very misinformed and sometimes even scared of people on dialysis. Outrageous as it sounds, you may run across a co-worker (although they may be afraid to say it out loud or to you directly) who is most certainly wondering, "Is dialysis contagious?"

This begs the question of whether you should share your medical situation with your colleagues. There really is no easy answer to this question and the quickest response would be, it depends. First of all, do your colleagues *need* to know? Sometimes because of your dialysis schedule you may need to do a little explaining in order to avoid unnecessary resentment as to why you are receiving what they may feel is preferential treatment. Or, if you are on a transplant list you may need your colleagues to be informed of certain projects in case you have to take a sudden leave and unexpectedly put them in charge. However, in some situations your co-workers really may not *need* to know about dialysis provided you are getting your work done and they are marginally or not at all affected.

Second, you may want to contemplate whether you *want* your colleagues to know about your renal failure and for what reasons. If it is your first day on the job and you find yourself telling anyone and everyone that you are on dialysis, stop and reflect about why you want this attention. However, if over time, you form a close camaraderie with specific co-workers you may feel that your renal failure is a part of you that you are comfortable sharing. While dialysis does not define you, it is after all a part of your identity.

Most important, if you've already proven yourself to be a capable worker and colleague, sharing the fact that you are on dialysis can be the best possible way to shatter many of the misperceptions that are so prevalent among friends and co-workers. Some of the reasons these old-fashioned stereotypes around dialysis and dialysis patients persist are because dialysis patients are not always visible. The more people who are on dialysis and are doing well choose to make it known that they are on dialysis, the more likely it is that these perceptions will change. So you do have an opportunity to make a positive difference, influence members of our society, and ascribe a more accurate face to what someone on dialysis looks like. This is a lofty responsibility that certain individuals are not comfortable with. Whether you want this responsibility to teach others is entirely your choice.

Last, you will likely find yourself in a number of work situations that you might not be able to fully participate in such as pizza parties, ice cream socials, or even happy hours—none of which are particularly healthy options for a person on dialysis. You may think, well, I'm better off just skipping the event entirely than having to hear people say, "Hey you're thin; how come you don't want any pizza?" or "You've barely touched your drink and we're already on our third round; don't you like your beer?" Having a fail-safe answer that you can fall back on while not having to go into a ton of detail will make these situations far less stressful to deal with. And it will keep you from feeling like the perpetual odd man or woman out. Participating in as many things you can that you find enjoyable is critical to your health. So if you enjoy hanging out with your colleagues don't skip these events. Instead, when and if a question comes up, just pull out your stock answer such as, "I'm on a special diet for health reasons." Most people will have enough common sense not to press further but if they do you can always say, "It's really not worth going into right now," and then swiftly change the subject to the latest in sports news or office politics. That will nicely but firmly indicate that you don't want to discuss it further.

The Alternative: Disability or Retirement

As we said earlier, some people really cannot work after going on dialysis. For example, we met the wife of a patient had worked for years as a cross-country truck driver. After going on dialysis he simply could not wed his demanding driving schedule to his equally demanding dialysis schedule. His best alternative at the time was to apply for disability. This can be very tough on a person emotionally and financially, but people are remarkably resilient and eventually patients do adjust. And just because you do not go to a job every day does not mean you can't volunteer or be involved in your community. There are so many opportunities to give back, even when on dialysis, that going on disability doesn't necessarily mean resigning yourself to sitting on the couch all day. As one woman on dialysis told us, "I hate to see people just go home and stay around the house all day. That will kill you. You need to get a life and get involved. I work at food banks and help senior citizens who are housebound. I take them to their doctor's appointments, help them around the house, take them shopping, sit and talk with them. Do like I do. Go help someone who is *really* sick. Or if you don't want to do that, volunteer at a library." To identify volunteer opportunities that meet your needs you can start by checking the yellow pages and contacting nonprofit organizations in your area. Or if you have access to the web, a few excellent sites with volunteer opportunities are listed below:

www.volunteermatch.org
www.idealist.org
www.volunteer.gov

Occasionally individuals will go on disability for a short time and then return to the workforce at a later date. However, once a person makes the financial transition to a less prosperous lifestyle it can be difficult to re-motivate and return. Although not technically on disability at the time, Maria was an example of someone who returned to the workforce after living as if she were on disability for a year. However, it took a significant amount of discontent to motivate her. In addition, she was a twenty-year-old with potentially more energy than a forty-year-old or sixty-year-old. If you go on disability and later decide to rejoin the workforce, you will need to justify the gap in your work history, which can be tricky and may make finding work a challenge. In some cases a decision to go on disability is clear. But in the event your case is not so clear-cut—for all these reasons—think very carefully before selecting to go on disability. You can of course return to work later, but keep in mind that you will likely have a steeper hill to climb to get there.

Or perhaps instead of disability you are on the cusp of retirement or have already passed sixty-five and can retire immediately and receive a pension. Depending on your age, retirement may be an alternative to disability, although, you may also want to consider still working in some capacity such as volunteering just to keep busy and active. Do you have to retire at sixty-five? No, not necessarily. These days many individuals continue to work beyond sixty-five. Daniel is one such individual who chose to continue working well past that age. In fact, when he was diagnosed with kidney failure at sixty-nine he continued to work full-time for many years and still continues to work part time. Now that you are on dialysis, you are not required to retire, although you may decide that you want to.

Practicalities of Finances and Insurance Plans while on Dialysis

Obviously decisions around disability and retirement are not only based on your physical and mental health but also on how these changes will impact you financially. And by financially we are not only referring to the paycheck that you draw but also to the health insurance benefits that you receive depending on your income and whether or not you are employed. Understanding the different types of health insurance coverage for dialysis patients and how that may affect you is a fairly complex topic, but we'll do our best to cover the basics. Then we'd recommend you follow up with your social worker to determine which health insurance options are available to you and which will serve you best.

Understanding Medicaid and Medicare

Let's start with a basic description of Medicaid, what it is, and who is eligible to receive it. Medicaid is a state-run program that receives federal funding. It is a form of insurance with extremely low co-pays associated with dialysis, doctor visits, hospital visits, prescriptions, and so on. There are two groups of people that qualify to receive Medicaid. One group is families with young children at home that meet low income guidelines. The other group is individuals who are over sixty-five or are blind or otherwise disabled and who meet low-income guidelines. Under the criteria set forth by the Aid to the Aged, Blind, and Disabled (AABD) program, individuals with renal failure are considered disabled. The low-income guidelines will vary from state to state but in general they are fairly rigorous and are de-signed to grant Medicaid to those individuals who truly must survive on small incomes. Many of the people who fall within this category may have previously been working for minimum wages, for sporadic periods of time, or for cash. Oftentimes they have been uninsured for much of their past working lives. Ironically, now that they have renal failure and can qualify for both disability and Medicaid, they may suddenly find themselves in much better financial situation than they had been in previously.

Although this is good news for these individuals, it can also be an eventual catch-22 should they want to seek gainful employment and get off disability. If, for example, they return to the workforce and begin to earn enough money that they no longer fall within the low-income guidelines, they will often no longer be eligible for Medicaid. And even though they are earning more, their health care premiums will rise and their out-of-pocket expenses will increase. Overall, going back to work may not be cost effective for them, so in many cases, staying unemployed is the better financial option. Some states, in an effort to help individuals return to work without being penalized financially, will offer Medicaid buy-in programs. This means that for a nominal fee these individuals can still receive Medicaid and the low costs associated with it.

Medicare, on the other hand, is a health insurance program that is paid out of a federal reserve of social security funds. Throughout our lives as we work, we pay social security taxes and if we work a minimum number of years, we become eligible to qualify for Medicare. In some cases an individual may also be eligible to qualify for Medicare through a spouse's work history. Provided you or your spouse has put in the necessary amount of time to be eligible, for you to then qualify to receive Medicare you must either be over sixty-five or disabled at any age. And similar to Medicaid, if you are on dialysis, you are considered by Medicare to be disabled. If you begin peritoneal or home hemodialysis, Medicare can go into effect immediately. If, however, you begin with in-center hemodialysis Medicare coverage does not go into effect until ninety days after your first treatment.

On a historical note, in 1972 Congress passed an amendment mandating that Medicare cover the costs of dialysis and this coverage went into effect July 1, 1973, thus ensuring that from then on in the United States dialysis would be available for all who needed it. Before then, because of the limited supply of dialysis machines, individuals were deemed either to receive or not receive dialysis by medical panels. Thus this was earth-shattering legislation for Americans with kidney failure.

As of 2005, Medicare now has a prescription drug program. For the most part, this is good news for dialysis patients, as most of the drugs that dialysis patients need are covered. There are some cases when one brand of drug is covered while another is not, but this is more disruptive to the medical staff than it is to the patient. Even with this plan, the numbers of drugs an individual must take multiplied by the cost of co-pay per drug per month can be very expensive and at times unaffordable for patients on fixed monthly incomes. Dialysis patients are eligible for some medication financial assistance programs, which we will talk about shortly.

Medicaid and Medicare both cover a percentage of fees associated with mental health services as well as physical health services. This includes visits to psychiatrists, psychologists, and social workers. However, many mental health providers have small practices that are not equipped to deal with the paperwork required by Medicaid and Medicare and for this reason will often charge a comparable sliding-scale fee that a patient then pays out-of-pocket. If you need to see a good mental health professional, ask up-front what his or her insurance and payment policies are. If the person's services are not covered, often he or she will refer to professionals whose fees are funded.

Private, State, and Medigap Health Insurance Plans

Every private health insurance plan is different and individuals who have a private health insurance plan through an employer may initially opt not to apply for Medicare depending on the specific costs, premiums, co-pays, and flexibility of their plan. However, there is a federal law that protects private insurance companies from having to cover dialysis costs indefinitely. The law essentially caps the amount of time (currently two and a half years) these private insurance companies must pay for dialysis before Medicare must be employed to cover the costs. When starting dialysis you should meet with your social worker to understand if you might be best served to stick with your private insurance initially and move to Medicare later on, or if you would be better served by moving to Medicare immediately. You will want to look at which solution will save you the most money, as well as which will enable you to be treated by the doctors or centers that you want.

In either case you may also choose to keep both insurance policies working for you, one as your primary insurance and the other as your secondary insurance. Of course, after two and a half years, Medicare must become your primary insurance. At that point you can either keep your private insurance policy as a secondary insurance plan or you can drop it entirely. As we said, every private insurance plan is different depending on your annual out-of-pocket premiums and co-pays, so you'd be very wise to spend time with your social worker to understand what will be the least expensive option for you.

Many states have health laws that give individuals with chronic illnesses better health insurance options than those available through private insurance companies. If your state has such an option, you may want to investigate the benefits of carrying this insurance.

Last, as we mentioned, in-center hemodialysis coverage under Medicare goes into effect only ninety days after the first treatment. And for all dialysis patients, Medicare covers only a percentage of the total treatment costs. This is the primary benefit to having a secondary insurance policy—either private or state—to help cover some or all of the costs that are not paid through Medicare. In addition, there is a third alternative that can assist with these costs: Medigap. There are several different Medigap policies but they all serve the same purpose: to help you with the monetary "gaps" that Medicare does not cover. Like private and state health care plans, you will pay a premium for a Medigap policy.

Other Forms of Financial Assistance

Maria mentioned that there were educational grants available to her because she was on dialysis. We discussed this with our expert social worker and she told us that there are several foundations and nonprofits that can help dialysis patients pay for a whole host of expenses associated with dialysis such as medications, the first ninety days of in-center hemodialysis treatments that are not covered by Medicare, and educational or vocational training, among others. And she advised, "Don't try to figure it out all by yourself. There are questions you don't even know to ask and there are resources that exist that would never occur to you. Speak with your social worker, nurse, or dietician about your concerns. Many times there are solutions or at least possibilities of solutions that you wouldn't have the slightest idea about. Using the professionals around you to find these resources is very important."

As an example you may not know that every state has an office of rehabilitation services. These offices are designed to assist people who have a variety of physical and mental disabilities to optimize their work abilities and opportunities. They can provide training or give you money toward technical courses, or a GED or bachelor's degree. If you are disabled these services are entirely free. Most of the time they can be extremely helpful, but occasionally you may encounter a rehabilitation counselor who is misinformed and thinks dialysis patients are unable to work. But you don't have to accept no for an answer. If you have an idea of what you want to do and you just need somebody to help you get there, these offices have the resources to help. And although there are many people on dialysis who are able to continue working in highly physical vocations, there are some who find they no longer have the strength and endurance to continue in their field. For these people, the rehabilitation services offices can be particularly helpful. Rather than going on disability indefinitely, such individuals, with the help of vocational rehabilitation assistance, can many times re-train themselves to do alternative types of work.

A Job Well Done

At the end of the day, most of us like to feel a sense of purpose and meaning. We take joy in our accomplishments, which sometimes include performing a task or a job for pay, for intellectual stimulation, for companionship, or for the pure joy of helping others. Now that you find yourself on dialysis, your professional life will likely shift a bit to accommodate dialysis. You may need to redefine exactly how, when, and where you find your sense of purpose and meaning. But rest assured, you need not plan on relinquishing every bit of your time to dialysis. And if you are lucky, you may even be able to continue doing what you were doing before you started dialysis. Even if your world tips upside down temporarily, it will likely right itself eventually and it need not come to a complete and permanent halt. Remember to allow yourself the time to be sick and to feel better. Then once the worst has passed, try to go back to doing what you normally did—or as close to it as you can get. That, unto itself, will be a job well done.

Nine

Adapting to the Dialysis Diet, Curbing Liquids, and Embracing Exercise

EARLIER IN THE book we explained at length why it is so important to follow the dietary and liquid guidelines put forth by your physicians. First, your willingness and ability to follow the rules can impact how long you are on this earth. And if that is not enough to motivate you, bear in mind that what you eat or drink and how much of it will directly affect how good or bad you feel before, during, and in between your dialysis sessions. OK, you are probably thinking, "I want to follow the rules, but sometimes sticking to them is easier said than done." And you may have a point. Many of us know that flossing is good for our gums, but do we do it every day? How many of us smoke even though we know it is terrible for our health? Sometimes we *want* to do better, we fully understand the implications of our actions, and yet we continue to practice bad habits and make poor choices. This is the challenge that many dialysis patients struggle with. We understand it is very difficult for some people to adapt to and comply with the diet and the fluid restrictions. Oh, do we understand! And that is why this chapter is less about guilting you into doing what is right than it is about empowering you to take control and giving you the tools to help you make smart choices when it comes to diet and exercise.

For the most part peritoneal dialysis patients are less restricted than hemodialysis patients when it comes to food and drink. This chapter may still be of interest to PD patients but will likely be more relevant to patients on hemodialysis.

For a chapter with tips on diet and exercise for dialysis patients, who better to jump-start the discussion than a dietician at a dialysis clinic? Susan sat down with Julie, a dietician who had been working with dialysis patients for over eight years. This was a prime opportunity for Susan to learn just what made dialysis patients tick when it came to curbing their diet and liquid intake. What motivated them to do well? Alternatively, what kept them from making the changes that would make them feel better? Julie was happy to share her insights into what she had learned over the years from so many of the patients she had worked with.

Julie's Story, a Dietician's Perspective

Do you find that people struggle with the diet?
"Yes very much so. You have two groups of patients. One group of patients never really learned about a healthy diet growing up and they just want to eat what they grew up eating. They are struggling because everything they like is off limits. Then you have another group that learned to follow a healthy diet and suddenly they are struck with this task of limiting foods that they previously thought were healthy. So whether or not you were following a healthy diet before dialysis you still have to make big changes."

What motivates your patients to stick with the diet and limit their liquids?
"The most effective motivation is usually a three-part process. First I try to get them to change something. Once they make the change they will see some improvement. Then I congratulate and praise them on that improvement. Most patients are motivated by

praise and positive reinforcement. I will also try to make it difficult for them to come up with an excuse for why they can't make it happen. We are all guilty of thinking up excuses for why we don't want to do something. But I try to stay positive and focus on the positive. For example, when someone starts on dialysis sometimes I'll give them a grocery list of the foods that they *can* have as opposed to a list of what is off limits."

Julie explains that this is an ongoing process of motivation and education for the patient. Most lab tests are done monthly but some can be done weekly. For example, if a patient's phosphorous levels are quite elevated he or she would be retested a week later. Perhaps the patient had initially forgotten to take a binder or had eaten something that he or she did not realize was so high in phosphorous. Hopefully, if the patient were to be very careful the following week, he or she would see an immediate improvement to the phosphorous levels after being retested. What is helpful for patients is that they can receive feedback early and often. Julie views her role in this process as educator. She can use the lab results to explain to patients and their families how specific foods and or medications can directly impact the values that appear on the printout. Julie then elaborated on why certain patients are able to succeed at making changes to their dietary lifestyle while others are not.

What are the key characteristics of patients who do well on dialysis?

"I think the patients that do well are the ones who feel that they have some control. If patients feel that they can alter what they eat or drink and actually enhance their health and improve their life then they are easier to work with. They will listen, be open to suggestions, try them out, and let you know if the suggestions worked. The patients who are willing to explore what it will take to feel better are the ones who, in my eyes, do better."

What are the key characteristics of patients who don't do well on dialysis?

"I think perhaps patients who have a lack of self-confidence do not do as well. These patients feel like they don't have that much control over their actions. I suspect some just feel they are destined to be unhealthy and there isn't anything they can do to feel better. Likewise, they feel that they don't have the capability to control what they eat. I often hear patients say, 'I don't have willpower.' They assume that they can't do any better, and that is simply not true. But it *will* be true as long as they feel that they don't have the power to change what they do."

So basically you are saying that attitude can have a big effect on their ability to make dietary changes?

"Yes. I strongly feel that if people believe they can make a difference in their lives, then they will. The people that really say to themselves, 'Ok, I can do this. I can do better. I can do this to protect my heart. I can do this to protect my bones.' These are the people who are going to thrive on dialysis."

How important a role do the immediate family members play?

"I think family plays a huge role. There are a lot of ways that a family can help or hurt a patient. You don't want someone trying to sabotage what you eat. That can be very harmful. On the other hand, many families are very devoted to learning about the diet and trying to shop and cook for it. Often when patients get their lab reports I'll jot notes on the paper for them to share with their families. A lot of times they will say to me, 'My family really likes to see this' or 'I always share this with my family.' "

What are your thoughts on cheating?

"I think people should enjoy the foods that they like. I'm not a stickler for *never* having pizza or *never* having a piece of cheesecake. There are certain foods that are worth eating to that person and that person should eat those foods on rare occasions and in small amounts. I would encourage cheating when it is planned. For example, if you know you are going to eat enchiladas that day, be very careful the rest of the day; take your pills with you and savor every little bit of your meal like it was your last enchilada. I think to occasionally eat something you know is a forbidden fruit, but to eat it in such a way that you do not overindulge, is important. This can really give you a lot of self-confidence in your ability to stray without entirely losing control and still be OK."

Have you ever contemplated what it would be like to be on dialysis?
"I do think about it all the time. I think it would be very hard to sit still for so long without wiggling. I'm a wiggler. But I think getting that report that tells you how you are doing would be very motivating for me. Even now, I like getting tests back on how my cholesterol is. I suspect that even the folks who don't appear to be as interested in their reports, deep down inside they also like to hear when they've done well. The reports show that everyone has the potential to do something positive for his or her life."

Let's say you are motivated to make changes, you do believe in yourself, and you have enough self-esteem to take care of yourself. You are committed to taking charge and refuse to resign yourself to helplessness. Excellent! You are off to a great start. Clearly, according to Julie, these are the philosophical cornerstones to success. Then what? What do you need to do to make it happen? The rest of this chapter will be chock full of practical suggestions that pertain to the dialysis dietary and fluid restrictions. We'll also include some suggestions about kicking up your heels and incorporating exercise into your life.

Eating Right

A Brief Refresher: What's in It for Me?

Most people on dialysis will need to follow a low phosphorous, low potassium, low-sodium, high-protein diet. Wow! That sounds like a lot to keep up with. But don't be overwhelmed. Plenty of folks do it and you can too. We've touched on many of these dietary restrictions earlier in the book, but let's do a very quick review plus add a bit more information about them. We'll briefly explain the importance of each restriction and how it affects your body.

Phosphorus: Now that your kidneys aren't working properly, phosphorus can build up in your blood, and this causes calcium in your blood to drop. This in turn causes your parathyroid glands to become too active. Over time, this overactivity creates a loss of calcium from your bones and eventually weakens them. You can protect your bones by cutting down on foods high in phosphorus and by taking phosphate binders (which prevent phosphorus from being absorbed in the blood) and supplements like calcium and vitamin D. High-phosphorus foods include all dairy products like milk, ice cream, and cheese, or foods made with a lot of dairy products, such as waffles and pancakes. Additional high-phosphorus foods include dried beans and peas (with the exception of green beans), nuts and peanut butter, and beverages such as cocoa, colas, and beer.

Potassium: Potassium keeps your heartbeat regular and your muscles, including your heart, working right. Like phosphorous, potassium levels are typically regulated by the kidneys. Now that yours are no longer working properly, your potassium levels may increase. If your potassium levels become too high you are at risk of having a heart attack. Your lab reports will identify whether your potassium levels are safe, concerning, or dangerous. You can lower your potassium levels by cutting back on foods such as bananas, cantaloupe, oranges, avocado, spinach, tomatoes, and many other foods that are high in potassium.

Sodium: Sodium, known in common language as salt, makes us retain fluid. And it makes us thirsty. Aside from table salt, it is also found in large amounts in canned soup and vegetables, pizza, pretzels, pickles, and processed meats such as hot dogs, salami, bacon, and cold cuts. Limiting sodium, which minimizes fluid intake and retention, may create less stress on your heart, make it easier for you to breathe, help keep your blood pressure under control, and make your dialysis treatments more comfortable.

Protein: Protein plays a critical role in promoting muscle growth and tissue repair. Protein from your tissue, as well as protein that you eat, is broken down to urea that accumulates in the blood and is removed by dialysis. In order to make up for this loss of protein you will need to eat larger quantities of high-quality protein that is usually found in eggs, fish, chicken, and meat.

Food Glorious Food

That's a lot of restrictions to keep track of and, yes, you are going to have to make some big changes to your diet, but a key element to your success will be constantly reminding yourself that you can still have so many delicious foods. Before or immediately after starting treatment, you will receive a list of good and bad foods from your dietician or doctor. Over time you will come to know this list by heart, but initially take it with you to the grocery store, to restaurants, and to other people's homes and refer to it frequently. Try to treat the diet as an opportunity to explore and discover food anew. You may even uncover foods and food products that you never knew existed or barely ate before—foods you will now come to love. There will suddenly be foods that you need to eat more of, like chicken. And there will be foods that you'd otherwise imagine to be healthy that you must now eat very little of, like bananas. But in the end, you will still have plenty of nutritious and delicious options to choose from. And like Julie said, you might be best off focusing on the foods that you *can* eat rather than on the foods that you shouldn't eat.

One of the reasons it is important to focus on the positive is to avoid feeling deprived or cheated. Dialysis patients are like children when it comes to food. If you tell them they can't have something, they *immediately* want it! Better to focus on the food choices that are tasty, satisfying, and good for you. It may be hard to imagine at first, but in time you will get accustomed to your new diet and your taste buds may even adapt.

Living under the Same Roof: Eating by the Same Rules?

Julie touched on the importance of family members when it comes to adapting to the diet. As one gentleman reflected, "I think the diet is harder on my spouse than it is on me. She has to go in the closet to eat chocolate, orange juice, peanuts, and cheese. She has all of the things that I'm not supposed to have but she is very supportive and does it behind my back." As you can imagine, if you are surrounded by individuals who are encouraging you to eat ice cream and pizza with them, that would be extremely unhelpful and disruptive to your success. On the other hand, now that you must give up, or at the very least minimize, your consumption of certain foods, is it fair to expect other family members to do so as well? What is their role in all of this? Do they need to become closet eaters?

If you live under the same roof, your family members' habits and willingness to be supportive will have a profound effect on your success as well. Let's be clear: as Julie mentioned, it is extremely important to have your family members fighting the good fight with you. But you'll need to find a happy medium that is both helpful for you and not overly limiting for them. Perhaps you can agree to only keep foods in the house that are good for you, or that you do not care about. For example, let's say you've never really cared for oranges, but your spouse loves them. As a dialysis patient, oranges aren't very good for you, but they aren't particularly tempting either. There is no reason your spouse shouldn't have oranges stocked at home. On the other hand, what if your Achilles heel is Cookies and Cream ice cream? If you get as close as a country mile to a pint of that stuff you just can't resist. Well then, it wouldn't be very supportive for this to be in your freezer. Perhaps in this case, your family can save their consumption of ice cream for separate visits to Baskin & Robbins.

The key to your family members' support is education. Just like you, they must familiarize themselves with the list of foods high in potassium, phosphorous, and salt. They must take the time to understand what is good for you versus what is bad for you. The dialysis diet is often anti-intuitive. What may seem healthy to most people may be very unhealthy for a dialysis patient. If your family members do not reeducate themselves about what *really* is healthy for you, they may try to be helpful but unknowingly undermine your efforts to eat well. For example, one patient told us that her mother was always saying to her, "You are too thin, you need to eat more. You need to keep up your strength." The woman's mother would then proceed to push foods on her daughter that clearly weren't good for her to eat. While the patient's mother had the right intentions, she didn't understand the dialysis dietary restrictions well enough to follow through correctly and instead was unknowingly sabotaging her daughter's efforts.

Following good intentions with bad recommendations can be easily remedied with a little education. If you feel that you aren't up to the task of educating your family members, perhaps arrange for a consultation with the dietician and ask your family to attend with you. When you get your lab reports back and have done well or shown improvement, involve your family members too. Show them how well you are doing! Like you, they also enjoy positive feedback and whether it is a conscious decision on their part or not, their willingness to support you is also reflected in those lab numbers.

Dining Out

Many of us enjoy being able to eat out with friends or family, plus it is a treat not to have to cook or clean up after a meal at home. Dining out is often a fun, social affair. But stepping out of the house, away from our own kitchen, means that we have more rather than fewer choices. With the increase in selection comes an increase in unhealthy options. The key to success when dining out is planning ahead. By following the suggestions below you can still eat out in a healthy manner:

- If you are planning to eat a meal out, let's say dinner, try to be extra careful with your intake during the morning and the afternoon. Throughout the day save your fluids and eat smaller portions of foods low in sodium, potassium, and phosphorus.

- You can really eat anywhere, but some restaurants will have more healthy selections than others. Look for restaurants and cuisines that will give you the most to choose from, but know that if you end up someplace with fewer choices, there will always be *something* for you to eat.

- If you saw the movie *When Harry Met Sally*, you'll recall that without fail, every time Sally ordered off a menu she'd ask for substitutions and special preparations. When it comes to ordering food the way you want it, don't be shy; be a Sally. These days most restaurants are accustomed to serving diners with dietary constraints. Feel free to ask for sauces and dressings on the side. Don't hesitate to ask for ingredients to be left out or for substitutions to be made. Basically using the menu as a guide, design a meal that you'd like to eat and will be good for you. Then place your order. Provided you aren't asking the chefs for an extra cross-town trip to the market, you'll be surprised at how often (almost always) they are able and happy to accommodate you.

- Try to stay away from fast-food chains. Aside from being very high in fat, fast foods are typically very high in sodium as well. If you just can't resist, then ask for the nutritional content information of the menu items, which most fast-food restaurants can provide. Then make the best informed choice. Opt for kid-size portions and request that your items be prepared without salt.

- When ordering from any restaurant, try to avoid spicy foods as they tend to make you thirstier.

- Ethnic restaurants are often excellent options for dialysis patients. There are many healthy selections to choose from at

Indian, Korean, Japanese, and Mediterranean restaurants, just to name a few.

- Following this ethnic train of thought, if you live in a town or city that has a sizable Jewish population, find out if there are any nondairy kosher restaurants nearby. Nondairy kosher restaurants, meaning restaurants that use zero dairy in their recipes, are a great option for dialysis patients. Even if something on the menu appears to be made with dairy, it is actually made with a substitute and is entirely dairy free.

- Splitsville is a good place to visit when you are on dialysis. Most dieticians will agree that the food portions in America have grown to ridiculously unhealthy sizes. Consider splitting meals with a friend or family member or, when you order, ask the waiter to bring half of the meal and put the other half in a container to go. That way you won't be tempted to overeat. Or, for portion control, order an appetizer as a main dish.

- Last, bring your binders with you and take them as needed. In fact, keep binders conveniently on hand anywhere that you might find yourself eating, in or out of the house. One patient told us that since going on dialysis he has learned to keep binders in his truck, car, wife's purse, and bedside table.

Holiday Eating

Aside from dining out, the next big challenge for many of us to stick to our dietary guns is often holiday eating. Much of what we recommended above also applies to holiday eating but here are a few additional tips:

- Try to eat a small meal of healthy foods before partaking in a holiday feast. This way you'll be less inclined to overindulge in foods that aren't as healthy for you.

- Both white and sweet potatoes can be used in a variety of dishes provided they've been peeled and soaked overnight in a bowl of water. Potassium is leached out of the potato and into the water, leaving behind a potato that is good for you to eat!

- Good food choices during traditional American holidays are beef, turkey, fresh fish, rice, noodles, pasta, white bread stuffing, green beans, and apple, cherry, and mixed berry pies. Poor food choices are ham, potatoes and sweet potatoes that have not been soaked, pumpkin or pecan pie.

Creativity in Cooking and Shopping

In addition to tips for dining out and holiday eating, we've discovered a few other gems as we've embarked on this new culinary adventure:

- Natural or organic grocery stores like Whole Foods or Wild Oats are excellent places to find dialysis-friendly products and canned goods. They have many foods and drinks that have low or no preservatives, which often means low sodium or low potassium. But of course, the critical test is to read the label.

- The best cookbook that we've seen written specifically for individuals on dialysis is titled "Cooking for David: A Culinary Dialysis Cookbook." For the most part, the recipes are easy, use common ingredients, and are quite tasty. Specifically for those who are first introduced to dialysis and are fearful of cooking within the confines of so many restrictions, this cookbook is probably the best place to get started.

- Once you've got a good grasp on the diet and have built up your culinary confidence, you can then experiment with just about any recipe in any cookbook. Margie has learned to take many of the recipes in her tried and true Better Homes & Gardens cookbook and adapt them, using common substitutions to meet Daniel's dietary needs. As an example, she frequently substitutes just a fourth of a cup of low-sodium tomato sauce for the two cups of tomato sauce called for in a recipe, and uses onions and green and red peppers instead of tomatoes when making spaghetti sauce.

- For the most part, cheese is off limits, but Brie cheese is not processed and is lower in phosphorus, making it a best-choice dairy product for those on dialysis. However, you still need to eat it in moderation. If you crave a rich and creamy cheese, you might want to splurge and eat an ounce of Brie.

- New food products are constantly being developed and brought to market. Your dietician will know about any new products that might be of interest to you given your renal dietary needs.

Cheating versus Eating Poorly

We've also learned a very valuable concept about living on dialysis: cheating is okay. Eating the foods you love is a very important part of living. If you love chocolate and you tell yourself, "Well now that I'm on dialysis I guess I'll never eat chocolate again," then you are living to dialyze instead of dialyzing to live. With that said, you now need to learn the importance of cheating in moderation. As Julie discussed, if you are going to cheat, you need to do it in a measured and controlled fashion as an occasional treat. You cannot go hog wild. Be judicious. But when you do cheat, you should thoroughly savor the experience. And after the fact, you can take pride in yourself for having allowed yourself to live a little without going crazy. Remember too, you can cheat occasionally, but if you find yourself cheating every day then you aren't cheating. You are just eating poorly.

How to Handle Liquid

Quenching Your Thirst

Some dialysis patients find adapting to the food restrictions to be the toughest challenge whereas others find limiting their liquids to be far worse. And some folks probably think these are equally miserable tasks. Regardless of which camp you fall into, you will probably have to make an effort at cutting back on how much you drink. In this section we'll briefly review the importance of minimizing your liquid intake. Then we'll share tips and tricks on making it happen.

Liquid: Less Is More

Why do dialysis patients need to cut back on liquids? We've explained this in great detail earlier in the book, but in brief, too much liquid is bad news. You've heard the old saying you are what you eat. For dialysis patients a more accurate statement would be, you are what you drink. Indeed, what dialysis patients drink literally stays with them between dialysis sessions, putting additional stress on all of their physical systems and creating both short-term and long-term complications and discomfort of varying magnitudes, including swelling, high blood pressure, shortness of breath, heart damage, cramps, dizziness, headaches, and nausea.

But what *exactly* is liquid, and what *exactly* is too much? Fluid is anything that flows, pours, or melts at room temperature. This includes water, milk, juice, coffee, tea, soft drinks, alcohol, ice, popsicles, ice cream, sherbet, soup, gelatin, yogurt, and pudding. And if you stop and think about it, you will realize that many fruits and vegetables, like lettuce, apples, or pineapple—while they cannot be poured—also consist in a large part of liquid.

Determining liquid weight gain is, as we discussed in Chapter 2, very much a process of trial and error. During the first few months of dialysis you will have to experiment to understand how much liquid you can consume between dialysis sessions to remain reasonably comfortable during and after your session. We've read in literature that the ideal weight gain is about two pounds per day. But most dieticians will tell you that there is no precise number that can be applied to everyone. The right amount of liquid weight gain varies by individual. With that said, you may want to start out with two pounds as a frame of reference. Check with your doctor or nurse as to how many recommended ounces of liquid a day you should be consuming to stay on track. Weigh yourself every day to see how you are doing. If you gain more than two pounds in one day that should serve as a warning that you are likely consuming too much liquid. Eventually you will become familiar with your body on dialysis and what is the optimal liquid weight gain for you. Bear in mind that if, as an example, you are on a Monday, Wednesday, Friday dialysis schedule you will always have gained more on Mondays because you will have gone the longest stretch without dialysis. This means that during your long stretch you should be even a little more aware and careful of your liquids than you would be during the rest of the week.

Now that you know what liquid is and how much is too much, we'll list a number of the helpful hints we've compiled over the years for beating the urge to drink too much and too often. Not all of these will work for you. The key is to try them out and seek out a few techniques that will likely help you cut down on your thirst, beat the heat, and minimize the discomfort of mouth dryness.

Quick Tips for Drinking Less

- Use small cups and glasses to give you the illusion that you are drinking more rather than less.

- Spread out your liquid consumption throughout the day by drinking small amounts more frequently rather than just having a few large portions two or three times during the day. This will help you feel more satisfied.

- Learn to sip instead of guzzle.

- When dining out asked the waiter not to refill your glass or ask him or her to remove it from the table altogether. This will ensure that you don't keep drinking unnecessarily.

- Add fresh lemon to ice cold water to help cut down your thirst.

- Consult with your doctor about drinking alcohol, but if you do choose to partake in an alcoholic beverage, avoid mixed drinks. Have it "on the rocks" or "straight up" to minimize liquid.

- Learn how to take pills with applesauce or use your liquid at meals to take your pills.

- Bring your own homemade low-sodium popcorn to the movies. You'll save both salt and money.

Quick Tips for Beating the Heat

- On hot days, serve up your drinks cold. Put them in a frozen mug or use plastic decorative ice cubes if you wish to avoid melted ice watering down your drink. You can use real ice cubes, but you'll need to factor them into your liquid intake.

- Likewise, you can suck on small amounts of ice or eat in moderation flavored crushed ice for variety. By sucking, you are essentially making your liquid consumption last longer.

- Suck on small amounts of frozen grapes.

- Stay inside and in the shade as much as possible.

Quick Tips for Relieving Dry Mouth

- Brush and rinse your mouth with cold refrigerated mouthwash.

- Chew sugar-free gum or suck on sugar-free hard candy.

- Suck on a lemon or lime.

- Snack on cold fruits or vegetables that are within your dietary allowance.

We've listed here just about every diet and liquid tool and trick we've heard of. Of course, you'll probably uncover a few others, but do test out some of the tricks above and if you find something that works, stick with it.

Get in Motion

Movers and Shakers: The Positive Impact of Exercise

We cannot simply talk about diet and health without also addressing exercise. In this day and age, our society has learned that the two go hand in hand. Exercise is good for your cardiovascular system, your waistline, your energy level, balance, flexibility, and your overall emotional and physical well-being. Just because you are on dialysis doesn't mean that you are exempt from starting an exercise routine. In fact, exercising may now be more important to your well-being than ever. Do check with your physician, however, before you get started on any exercise regime. Provided that you get the all-clear, you will have no excuse not to exercise. Moreover, you'll need to stick with an exercise routine. Many of us have the best of intentions when we start exercising, and a month later our intentions are nowhere to be found while we are planted firmly on the couch. With this in mind, your goal is to (a) get started and (b) keep going until (c) exercise becomes a part of your routine that you simply cannot do without.

How can one move from point (a) to point (c)? We will share with you a few suggestions to help you toward this end. Most of our exercise suggestions here are not specific to dialysis patients but are universal tips about exercise that are equally relevant to the dialysis community.

First, find something that you enjoy doing. Do you like to walk, ride a bicycle, swim, or take ballroom dance classes? The great thing about exercise is that there are so many types to choose from. Pick something that you like and start there. For example, if you hate jogging then don't force yourself to jog. Making yourself do something that you don't like is not a recipe for success. But if you like to walk, then make walking your exercise of choice. Chances are if you find enjoyment in your activity of choice, that will naturally encourage you to want to get out and do it more often.

Second, start out slowly and build up both your pace and overall time spent exercising. For example, perhaps you are overwhelmed at the thought of getting started. If that is the case, then just walking out the door the first time will be considered a success. Don't set unreasonable expectations for yourself. If you haven't exercised for weeks, months, or years, perhaps start out by walking for fifteen minutes at a leisurely pace. Over time, slowly add increments of five additional minutes to your walk until eventually you are up to thirty minutes. Likewise, perhaps start out exercising twice a week and slowly build up to three to four days a week. Then start working on increasing your pace. But don't overdo it in the beginning. If you set your sights too high and overexert yourself, you may find your workout overly strenuous and that may turn you off from continuing your routine. Remember, it's not where you start; it is where you finish.

Third, don't worry about what other people will think. Many of us avoid going to the gym because we are self-conscious or worried about what others might think of our too large or too weak or too slow or too uncoordinated physique. Forget what others think. If they knew what you were contending with, and on top of everything you have to do to stay healthy you've gotten yourself to the gym, they would think you are a star. And even if they didn't, they are too busy thinking about themselves to be passing judgment on you.

Don't be afraid to look foolish in other people's eyes. Just try your best and get out there.

Fourth, sometimes it is easier to get over our inhibitions and inertia by having an exercise buddy. Also an exercise buddy will force you to continue exercising on days when you don't feel very inspired. Sometimes just knowing that you have to be accountable to another person ensures that you will show up and participate when you might otherwise be inclined to settle in on the couch. So forge a partnership with a friend, a child, or a spouse and encourage each other to create and stick to a routine. You might want to seek out a class at your local YMCA, community center, or athletic club. Many fitness centers or clubs have an extensive menu of classes to choose from for all ages, interests, and fitness levels. And for those who can afford it, a personal trainer once a week is also a fantastic investment in your health. A trainer will help create a routine that strengthens your body, and he or she will keep you motivated both during and between sessions.

Fifth, in addition to getting a cardiovascular workout, incorporate some weight training into your routine. Weight training works to strengthen and tone your muscles. You do not need to work out at a gym to do weight training. You can put together a program to strengthen your muscles just by doing a number of exercises at home. There are many videos and books that have detailed explanations of the types of movements that can strengthen your muscles.

Last, once you've settled into a routine, make sure to shake things up from time to time. Again, if you find that you are bored and are no longer having much fun with your exercise regime, then you will be more inclined to camp out on the couch. Adding some variety to your routine can renew your interest. For example, if you've been walking outdoors but have also always enjoyed bicycling, then try a local bike path one day just to see how you like it. If you do, then perhaps alternate between bicycling one day and walking the next.

If you've been exercising for years, then you'll know that nothing we've listed here is particularly new or earth shattering. These are simply practical tips that many fitness professionals have shared over time with the general population. Once you get in the groove you will really start to enjoy the many benefits that consistent exercise has on both your physical and mental well-being. And taking care of both body and soul is of critical importance to the overall health of a dialysis patient.

Patients Weigh In

In speaking with a number of patients, we heard a slew of comments about the dietary and liquid restrictions. As one patient told us, he and his wife have been known to refer to the dialysis diet as the "diet from hell." Other patients told us stories of terrible cramping from drinking too much liquid, or landing in the hospital from overindulging in watermelon. We heard about body aches and itching from eating too much phosphorous and not taking binders. We heard complaints that the binders are constipating. All in all, we heard that curbing desires for certain foods and liquids is tough.

Most of these same patients also told us that they have learned, albeit the hard way, how to say to themselves, "Enough. You have had enough." They have learned that certain foods and behaviors aren't worth the consequences. They have learned how to read the labels on food products at the grocery store. They have learned to retrain their taste buds. They have learned to soak their potatoes overnight if they want to make their favorite potato salad. They have learned that if they are going to eat ice cream or a slice of pizza then they must take their binders and be extra careful for the next few days. They have learned their limits. And even those who have learned all this, even they still claim that sticking with this diet and these limitations is sometimes *very* hard. Managing your diet and your liquids now that you are on dialysis probably won't ever become *easy*. But like many of the patients we've spoken with, you can learn to give it your best. Your body *will* respond positively to your careful attention. Oddly enough, this response will, in a sense, be a show of gratitude to you for your efforts. Or in simpler terms, eat well, drink little, and be merry; your body will thank you for it.

Ten

Traveling and Planning for Emergencies while on Dialysis

Taking a Leap of Faith

The world is a book and those who do not travel read only a page.
—*St. Augustine*

WHETHER YOU INTEND to read one page or twenty, you may feel that your world has suddenly shrunk now that you or a family member has gone on dialysis. You may even feel that you cannot travel beyond a thirty-mile radius of your dialysis clinic or your home. Whatever boundaries you've created in your mind, in most cases they are just that—boundaries of the mind. With some courage, planning, smarts, and a general belief in the kindness of others you can take your show on the road. In this chapter we will present a great deal of practical information that we've learned over the years about traveling while on dialysis. We'll also address common fears dialysis patients may have about travel and uncover some realities that will help to assuage these fears. Generally speaking we've found travel to be liberating and exhilarating. Above all, a trip away, an adventure, serves as a powerful reminder that life is meant to be lived.

Throughout the book we've shared the perspectives of several individuals who have encountered dialysis as either patients or professionals. Now it is time to share our own—or more specifically, Daniel and Margie's perspectives. At the time this book was written, Daniel had been on dialysis a little over seven years. When he began dialysis at the age of sixty-nine, he and Margie lived permanently in Illinois. All of their children lived far from them. Two of their three children lived in different states. The third lived across the Atlantic Ocean in London. Over the years Daniel and Margie's family expanded with the addition of several grandchildren. Eventually they had grandkids in California, Texas, and England. For many of the years that he was on dialysis, Daniel's mother was alive and living in Israel. His two brothers also lived in Israel. Margie's only sibling was in Washington, D.C. Clearly the world was not simply a book for Daniel and Margie. It was *the* book, the one that would record the happy occasions, celebrations, and milestones of their family. If they wished to share in many of these simple joys of life they would have to overcome any anxieties or uncertainties they had with regard to travel. Like the rest of the participants in this book, Daniel and Margie offered to be interviewed.

Daniel and Margie's Stories: Perspectives of a Traveler on Hemodialysis and His Spouse / Travel Companian

One spring day, Susan sat with her co-authors and parents at her home in Texas. At the time of the interview, Daniel and Margie had stopped to visit Susan's family in the midst of a driving vacation in the Texas Hill Country. Already having been in Fredericksburg and surroundings, they were essentially passing through, taking a prolonged pit stop in Austin before heading to Houston. Dialysis visits had been planned for months in advance and to date, had been going smoothly. Daniel and Margie were having a grand time. It seemed the perfect opportunity to hear what they had to say about stepping out in the world:

Can you tell me about the first time you traveled after Daniel began dialysis?

Daniel: "I went on dialysis June 20, 1999, shortly after undergoing a triple bypass on my heart. That following September we traveled for the first time. We went from Saturday morning to Monday morning so that I didn't have to dialyze away from home."

Margie: "We wanted to get away and needed a change of scene, but we were nervous about leaving the house. We drove to Lakeside, Michigan, which was only eighty miles from home, just to build some courage. It wasn't a great trip, but we do consider it a success. We walked around. We saw the lake. We tried to lift our spirits after Dan had been so sick."

What was your next trip? How did you choose your destination?

Margie: "Our next trip was two months later for Thanksgiving. None of our kids lived nearby and for special occasions and holidays we like to be where they are. That Thanksgiving we flew to California to see your sister and her family."

Daniel: "I went to a wonderful dialysis center in Mountainview, California. The staff was extremely receptive. Over the years, it has turned out to be my favorite clinic that I've traveled to because I've been there so many times. I'm as comfortable there as I am at my home clinic, even perhaps more comfortable."

What did you learn as you built on your successes, and began to travel more frequently and farther from your home?

Margie: "That first year, we traveled to Florida during peak tourist season and learned that when you go to a popular resort area at the height of the season you shouldn't expect to receive good dialysis times. The locals get the best times. Then the folks who live there for a few months in the winter get the second-best times. The short-term vacationers are left with the least desirable times."

Margie explains that while in Florida Daniel had to dialyze at 8 P.M. in a small town forty-five minutes away from the hotel. That meant she had to spend three hours in the small town by herself at night while he dialyzed. She ended up walking around a Target store at ten at night wondering who else—besides the wife of a dialysis patient—was shopping there at that time. She tells Susan that soon after that trip, she and Daniel went on a cruise where Daniel dialyzed in the evening. Again, this wasn't much fun for her. All the evening programs on the cruise were designed for couples, and she said she didn't fit in. Margie adds, "Eventually we learned how to best schedule Dan's dialysis times to fit when we want to be together. We now know that on a ship, morning dialysis is best. We can eat out and go to the shows together at night. But in an American city Dan can dialyze during the day or in the evening. There is a lot for me to do during the day. I can sightsee, shop, or walk. Or at night I can stay in the hotel and read. Evening dialysis is problematic if we are on a cruise or if the center is far from where we are staying."

Does a companion to someone on dialysis spend much of his or her vacation alone?

Margie: "Yes. Now when we go on vacation I spend about 40% of my vacation alone and I know how to do that quite well. But I am a very different person from the one I was when Dan first went on dialysis. I'm much more independent now. Initially I was used to doing everything with him, and I didn't know how to be alone. But the more I did on my own, the easier it became. I learned how to go to the movies alone. I love to window shop by myself. I'll go to museums, even plays. There are limitless opportunities for one to explore by oneself."

Does either of you get anxious or scared when you travel?

Daniel: "Every time I go to another city for dialysis, even if I've been there before, there is a certain amount of anxiety that comes over me. I always wonder, 'Will the people be nice? Will they be competent? Will everything work out all right?' I don't relax until the needle is in my arm and the dialysis starts. Going to a new place can be emotionally taxing, and I understand why some patients don't want to travel. But to my surprise, every time I arrive at a new clinic the staff anticipates that I will be nervous. As a result, they go out of their way to make me feel comfortable and at ease. To this day I've been to almost thirty clinics and the staff has responded this way every single time, everywhere, without exception. Some of my fellow patients have told me they don't travel, because they are afraid the clinics won't be good. I tell them, 'Don't worry about that. If you've known one dialysis clinic you've basically known them all.'"

Why do you travel?

Margie: "I think to see family and friends. At our age you want to see your children and your grandchildren. You want to celebrate the happy occasions that your friends have. If there are special occasions like weddings or graduations, it is very meaningful to me and to Dan that we aren't locked out of being able to go to these events and enjoy them. It is important that we can be like anybody else with our friends and family. But to experience these wonderful occasions, we had to build up our courage one trip at a time."

Daniel: "I think that one travels to cut through the monotony of life. This is true for people who are healthy too but when you are on dialysis the monotony is heightened and the schedule is exponentially tiresome. When you are on hemodialysis come rain or shine you have to go Monday, Wednesday, and Friday. You can't escape that cycle. Of course, even when you travel you still have to dialyze. But the change of scenery is good for the soul and adds color to your life. Whether you travel across the state, the country, or the ocean, you feel more alive, more like a normal person."

Margie: "A lot of times when we are someplace Dan will look at me and say, 'I can't believe I'm here *and* I'm on dialysis!'"

Daniel: "That's true. When I'm in a new place, I'll look around and say to Marge, 'My God, this is amazing! Here I am in the hills of central Texas walking along this small main street full of antique stores and I'm on dialysis—or, here I am in San Francisco at the Museum of Asian Art and I'm on dialysis!'"

Have you ever had a bad experience with dialysis when traveling?

Daniel: "No, not even Mexico, which some people think of as a third-world country. I've been to seven countries and to twenty different cities in the United States. I have *never* had a bad experience. I did have one marginally so-so experience when I was put on a faster dialysis speed than I was used to. It didn't agree with me. Now I've learned to tell the staff how fast I should be dialyzed when I go to a new clinic."

What role can a travel companion play in relieving the patient's anxieties?

Margie: "I'm very aware when we travel that Dan gets nervous. So I try to make his transition to a new place easier. I'll usually drive him to the clinic and pick him up. I try to be a calm, confident voice. I tell him it is going to be fine. I remind him of all the good experiences we have had. And when I walk into a clinic, I am a friendly soul. I always talk to the nurses and say 'Hi' to the other patients. I try to break the ice, warm up the place, so that Dan gets a nice welcome. I kid around. Friday when I dropped him off I said 'Have a good suds!' and all the nurses smiled. Basically, I try to smooth the way."

Daniel: "She does a very good job. She is an ambassador of goodwill."

Margie: "I haven't met a staff person who wasn't nice. When I leave, I will always say, 'Take good care of my husband!' I'll thank people for all their good care. People need to be appreciated. And I always, always smile. I never go into a clinic without a smile. I am very aware when I walk into a dialysis clinic that everyone there is fighting a battle."

Have you ever traveled on your own? If so, were you more nervous being alone?

Daniel: "Not really, because I traveled to places where my children or family lived so I knew I had support if I needed it. I went once to

Israel by myself and once to California. I wasn't worried either time. I think it would have been more difficult if I'd gone to a place where I hadn't known anybody."

Do you know other patients who travel?

Daniel: "Sure. Many patients travel. For example, there was a very gregarious, big fellow at my old clinic and his favorite summer pastime had always been fishing. When he first went on dialysis he thought he couldn't go fishing anymore and he was terribly upset. The people in the clinic told him, 'There is no reason you can't go fishing!' So he reluctantly and very nervously made plans to go to northern Wisconsin. He went for a week. When he returned he showed us all photos of the fish he caught. He was so incredibly happy. Every year thereafter he would take a fishing trip."

Daniel tells Susan that the most popular sites among fellow patients are Las Vegas, the Caribbean, Florida, and Alaska. Many dialysis patients travel for family occasions such as weddings, funerals, and baptisms. Even the patients who don't particularly like to travel will still make a big effort if there is a special occasion. He has known college students who traveled on spring break in Florida, an elderly couple who spent several weeks at a summer cottage in Michigan, and a retired businessman who returned to his native city of Belgrade for a month every year.

What advice would you give to someone who hasn't yet traveled while on dialysis?

Daniel: "My first piece of advice would be to get the initial anxiety out of your system. You will always have a little anxiety, but first you have to remove the big anxiety. Start with a short trip. Everything will go well, and then you can try a trip farther away. My second piece of advice would be that even if you don't have much money, travel. Go someplace inexpensive for a long weekend. Look around at the scenery and take a minute to think to yourself, 'Wow, look where I am. What an incredible experience.' Travel enriches life. I know that there are people who are really too sick to travel. I'm not recommending they travel. Rather, the persons who are rela-tively well, who are working and are leading a fairly normal life, they should travel."

How do clinics abroad differ from those in the United States?

Daniel: "For the most part, dialysis is really a universal treatment—although I've noticed that clinics in other countries are much more generous about providing food than those in the United States. I couldn't believe in Argentina they gave us cookies, juice, and cake! And in England they gave us an assortment of tea sandwiches, tea, and cookies. Certainly the *most* fun that I've ever had at dialysis was in Israel. It is the only place in the world where I really looked forward to going. The chairs are much closer to-gether so people can play chess, checkers, or cards and they have tremendous political arguments with each other. The time just flies there!"

Think back over the trips you've taken; what have been your favorites and why?

Daniel: "My favorite trip was the two-week cruise around Cape Horn from Buenos Aires to Chile. I enjoyed the experience of being on the sea a lot. When I first went on dialysis I didn't know this was possible. But I found out that most of the new, large boats offer trips with dialysis on board. For me, sailing and being on a ship was exhilarating."

Margie: "If I had to choose one trip, I'd say it has been this driving trip to Fredricksburg, Texas, and the Hill Country. It was like the old days when I was a child, and we'd get in the car and go. This trip was just the two of us, two kids on the road. But truthfully, for me, every trip has been a favorite because taking a trip is like normality. You don't let your illness own you. You are a person who just happens to be on dialysis. Traveling is not like beating the system. Traveling is like winning."

As the three sat together at Susan's dining room table, they fin-ished their conversation and moved on to an even more important topic of discussion: what to have for lunch. Susan turned off her tape-recorder and put away her notes. While she did so, she felt grateful that Daniel and Margie were willing to make the journey to her hometown time and again. She reflected on their adventure-some, courageous spirits, which had willed them onward despite the burdens of dialysis. Never before had Susan understood just how far Daniel and Margie have traveled in the past seven years. They hadn't simply crossed state lines and bodies of water; they had traversed their fears. And as with many travels that span a divide, theirs had transported them to an entirely new place.

Practical Suggestions for Travel and Emergency Preparedness while on Dialysis

The Fears That Ground Us

Daniel and many other dialysis patients do travel. In fact, so many travel that a cottage industry of companies with expertise in dialysis travel has emerged since the 1970s. Despite this, there are still many dialysis patients who choose not to travel. The reasons for this are varied. Some are simply too sick. Some may have never shown any interest or desire to travel before they were on dialysis. Some don't have the financial means to travel. But we have found that the most prevalent reason that dialysis patients don't travel is because they are afraid. Here are the top five travel fears that we've encountered:

1. When you show up to a new city, you might receive treatment in a shabby-looking neighborhood. And a shabby-looking neigh-borhood means that you won't get very good care.

2. The staff at a new clinic won't know what they are doing. They won't know you very well and therefore you will not receive the same level of care that you would get at your own clinic.

3. If you require urgent care in the case of an emergency you will be far from your doctors and your dialysis center. You will be in a bind.

4. When traveling you could possibly miss a flight due to bad weather, terrorism, or other reasons and actually get waylaid in another city without dialysis scheduled. Then what?

5. Actually locating and finding your way to a dialysis center in a new city or town will be difficult and stressful.

These fears are all very reasonable. As Daniel said, he has these fears every time he and Margie travel to a new place, but in reality these anticipated problems rarely materialize. Let's address these fears one at a time, explain what we've found to be the reality, and provide some tips on how to make sure traveling is not unduly stressful for you or a travel companion.

Facing Our Fears One by One

Fear Number 1: A shabby neighborhood will equal shabby care.

Ever hear the phrase "you can't judge a book by its cover?" This is quite true of dialysis centers. They are rarely located in fancy parts of town because of the high cost of real estate in these areas. Daniel once dialyzed in the sub-basement of a very old and dingy building in New York City. As he entered the building and descended to the bowels of the earth, he seemed to be headed toward a wreck of a center. As it turns out, the center, the staff, and his care were all first rate. You never know where you will land, but as you approach a new clinic try to view your visit as an adventure.

Fear Number 2: The staff won't know you and so they won't be able to provide the right or best kind of care.

As Daniel said, when you are new to a clinic as a traveler, the staff makes an extra effort to treat you well. They are extremely kind. This is true the world over. Also, it helps to be friendly and positive when you walk into a new clinic. This air of friendliness in combination with the staff's knowledge that you are nervous will result in their willingness to bend over backward to put you at ease. In addition, the social worker from your home clinic will, in advance, have faxed detailed treatment instructions to the staff at the new dialysis clinic. With these detailed directions on hand staff members are best equipped to mimic the care you would otherwise receive at home.

Fear Number 3: What if something out of the ordinary occurs with your health when you are far away? What then?

Well, the first thing to remember is that any major metropolitan area in the United States, and even much of the world, will have competent hospitals and good doctors. Depending on your circumstances you may be more inclined to travel to places where you have the security and comfort of knowing friends or family. That way, if a crisis occurs, you know there is someone you can lean on for help or for medical references. But what if you want to venture to a place where you don't have friends or family? In that case, you may be a little more comfortable having a travel companion, such as a friend, sibling, spouse, or child, who can go with you. That way if you need some extra care, you will have someone who can take charge or even just hold your hand while you are not feeling well. For example, when Daniel and Margie traveled to the Texas Hill Country they were a little bit off the beaten path. But if anything went wrong, Daniel had Margie as his backup.

Of course, if you are courageous enough you can step out on your own, without a travel companion, to a place where you know no one, and certainly many dialysis patients do. However, this will require suspending your fears and having faith that in the case of an emergency the people at the dialysis clinic will help you. Also make sure that family and friends know your travel plans and that the dialysis center has emergency contact names and numbers. The bottom line: whether you are traveling solo or with a buddy, in a place where you know somebody or nobody, you will need to figure out what your comfort level is. Plus you may see your comfort level grow as you become more accustomed to traveling. In the meantime, as you are building up your courage you might want to do what Margie sometimes does when she gets nervous. She silently hums these lyrics from *The King and I:* 'Whenever I feel afraid, I hold my head erect and whistle a happy tune so no one will suspect I'm afraid.' "

Fear Number 4: Travel hiccups such as flight cancellations or delays will interfere with dialysis and one's ability to stay healthy.

An Egyptian gentleman, who dialyzed alongside Daniel on one of the cruises, mentioned that he had been visiting his son in Phoenix on September 11, 2001. At the time he was scheduled to return to his home on the twelfth of the month. However, all the planes were grounded for at least a week. He said the dialysis center in his son's hometown was extremely helpful. They found him times to dialyze until flights resumed after a week and he could fly home. The point is, don't panic. Once you explain your situation, people will help you. Once, Daniel and Margie were to take a return flight from Austin to Chicago. They arrived at the airport to learn that all flights to Chicago had been cancelled due to poor weather. It was a Sunday night and Daniel was scheduled to dialyze the next day. They explained to the staff his situation and were told they could either fly to Wisconsin and drive to Chicago that evening or take the first flight out in the morning. Of course, Daniel and Margie worried "what if the flight is canceled tomorrow, what then?" but then they realized Daniel would be OK. If Daniel had to dialyze in Austin one more day, they were certain the center would not leave him high and dry. A center in town would find a place for him. As it turned out, the plane left the next morning as scheduled and Daniel dialyzed in his home center that afternoon.

Similarly when a flight from Boston to Chicago was overbooked, Daniel and Margie were told they had been bumped off the flight.

They explained Daniel's medical issues and were assured that he (although not Margie) would receive a seat. In that instance they asked immediately to speak to a manager. Their advice: if a travel crisis arises always stay calm, be nice, and if at all possible talk to whoever is in charge. As it turned out, they both made it on the flight.

Fear Number 5: You won't be able to find your way to a new center. You are on dialysis; you aren't brain dead. You can ask for directions and for help. If you are staying with family ask them to explain to you how to get from their home to the clinic, or to go with you if possible. If you are staying in a hotel ask an employee at the desk to help you arrange transportation and determine how long it may take to arrive or the best route to take.

Remember, every single time Daniel visits a new place and a new clinic he is scared and anxious before his first treatment. Until he finds his way and arrives at the dialysis center he thinks maybe he will get lost or maybe it won't be as nice as home. And every time, as soon as he arrives at the clinic and begins to receive care he doesn't know what he ever worried about. Margie uses humor to ease his fears and reminds him that they are on an adventure. Time and again his anxiety passes. Should you venture out, likely you will experience these same feelings, but remember many others have been there and done that. Take a deep breath and tell yourself you can do it too.

What to Know before You Go: Take Baby Steps First

Now that you have acknowledged your fears and have decided to get past them, what next? What do you need to do to begin traveling? First of all, start out slow and easy. One doctor told us that he tries to get all of his patients to start out by going away for a single night. He tells them not to worry about dialyzing away from home the first time they venture out. For many, just getting in a car and driving out of the area elicits a certain amount of anxiety. Once you've accomplished this, try dialyzing away from home. Perhaps go away for a long weekend where you have to dialyze only once. If possible, try visiting a place where you have friends or family. Then, if you are feeling increasingly comfortable, go away for several days. If you can afford it, perhaps even fly to a different destination and have several treatments away from home. With each trip you take your confidence in yourself and others will likely increase.

Travel on Peritoneal Dialysis, Home Hemodialysis, or while Awaiting Transplant

Daniel and Margie spoke from personal experience about travel while on hemodialysis. However, you can travel just as easily if you are on home hemodialysis or if you are awaiting a transplant. And if you are on peritoneal dialysis, travel is even easier in the sense that you don't have to plan your travels around visits to a center. Regardless of modality, you will just need to plan your travels accordingly. For those who are on home hemodialysis they will in most cases need to schedule in-center dialysis for the duration of their trip. There are instances of patients who have traveled with their own equipment by recreational vehicles (RVs) and have dialyzed at campsites with hook-ups for electricity. If you do not plan on dialyzing at a center, you should still contact a center before your trip and upon arrival so that they can be available to you for assistance if any issues or emergencies arise.

As we saw with Elena, a PD veteran in Chapter 3, you can absolutely travel while on PD. However, you will need to plan to have enough supplies for the duration of your trip. Depending on the length of your trip you may be able to take supplies with you or have them delivered to your destination in advance. If you are traveling within the United States, you need to arrange for delivery of supplies two to four weeks in advance. Check directly with your supplier regarding how much time they require. Outside of the United States you will need six to eight weeks' advance notice. Before leaving on your trip, call your destination to ensure that any supplies you have ordered for delivery have arrived. If using CAPD, you will need to account for a clean space where you can do your exchanges while traveling. If you are using CCPD, there are relatively small machines in existence that can be carried onto airplanes and used in hotel rooms or RVs. And again, even if you do not plan on stepping foot inside a dialysis clinic, you should still make arrangements with a local clinic to provide backup in the event of an emergency while you are away. Your social worker can help you to provide them with the necessary medical documentation or you may carry it with you.

Last, if you are awaiting a transplant you may also travel. However, you should first consult your transplant coordinator about any travel plans. Depending on your destination, you will either put yourself "on hold" temporarily while you are out of town, or you will provide a method of contact should you be close enough to return in time should an organ become available. In reality we find that many patients, as they get closer to the top of the transplant list, can still travel but often choose not to.

Plan Ahead

If you plan on traveling, the social worker at your clinic will become extremely important to you in the planning process. When you first start mapping out your trip, you'll need to provide your social worker with your itinerary. If there are several possible dialysis locations in the city, you may want to do a little bit of the legwork by going on the Internet and finding which one is closest to where you'll be staying. As a visiting patient you don't usually have much say over where or what times you receive your treatment. Basically, you take what you can get. However, if a specific time of day or a specific clinic is preferred, let the social worker know. That way he or she is aware of your preferences and can try to accommodate them.

The social worker then faxes all of your medical documentation (including recent lab results, electrocardiogram [EKG], chest x-ray, dialysis prescription, recent treatment records, etc.) in advance to clinics in the area of your destination and works to secure your dialysis schedule. These "away" clinics then inform your social worker if they can accept you depending on their availability. Typically you will need to work with your social worker no more than three months and no less than six to eight weeks in advance to schedule your dialysis. However, do inquire directly with your social worker as to how much advanced notice he or she suggests. Clinics in very popular vacation destinations during high travel seasons may be hard to get into. Before buying those nonrefundable airline tickets to Florida in January speak to your social worker. After researching, he or she may give you the green light. Alternatively, he or she may advise you to switch your itinerary or at the very least pay a little extra for the refundable tickets.

Get There Fast: Traveling for Emergencies

When Daniel's mother died, he needed to fly to Israel at a moment's notice to attend the funeral. Despite the lack of planning and lead time, the social worker was able to schedule dialysis treatments for him. Many dialysis centers will work very hard to accommodate patients in the event of a serious family emergency. Typically though, if you want to ensure that you have a dialysis spot and that you stay in the good graces of your social worker, you should plan nonemergency trips well in advance.

Learn the Financial Rules of the Road

Medicare covers 80% of the costs of dialysis while traveling in the United States. It does not cover any costs of dialysis outside the country. If you want to travel abroad or receive coverage for the 20% of in-state travel not covered by Medicare, you will need to procure a secondary insurance plan to pay for your dialysis sessions. One session itself can be in excess of several hundred dollars. Also many insurance plans require that you pay for the session up front and they will then reimburse you at a later date. You will need to determine how your insurance plan works, how much money you will have to pay up front, and how long it will take for you to be reimbursed. Daniel and Margie have always been reimbursed, but they have had to wait several months to receive payments. Medicaid will cover dialysis sessions only in the state where you live.

Hit the Road, Jack

For those who can't afford to fly, a driving trip may be just the ticket. You can cover a lot of ground and visit many interesting places in the United States. You will just need to plan your itinerary so that you are near a dialysis facility on the days that you will dialyze. One social worker we met with had scheduled dialysis for a patient who took a two-week driving trip the length of California. The social worker said it was fun to strategize and help with the dialysis planning portion of the trip. She worked to match the patient's wish list of destinations with a realistic timeline and itinerary that would land her at dialysis clinics in the right places at the right times. Remember that there are dialysis centers all over the country. However, some rural or out-of-the-way spots may not have a center nearby, but a little research and thoughtful scheduling can still make for a very enjoyable scenic tour.

Join the Crowd

There are many vacation packages that involve tours, and as individuals get older, many times they are more comfortable traveling in a group. This holds true for singles as well. You may be able to take an organized tour and opt out of the group activities during the times or days that you have to dialyze. One physician told us of a patient he treated who had loved to travel on tours prior to starting dialysis.

Afterward the patient desperately wanted to travel but was extremely self-conscious about her health and didn't want anyone to know that she was on dialysis. Her doctor was eventually able to convince her that the other participants on a tour wouldn't treat her oddly. As it turned out, the physician was right. The patient successfully overcame her inhibitions, resumed her travels, and although she had to sit out a few of the sights she no longer felt abnormal and unable to satisfy her love of travel.

Dialyze at Sea

As Daniel mentioned, there are many opportunities to dialyze on board major cruise lines. Dialysis usually takes place while you are at sea so that you can explore the ports of call. There is a nephrologist on board and on call for the entire voyage. Dialysis at sea allowed Daniel to travel to exotic destinations while dialyzing from a comfortable home base. He never had to be concerned about locating the dialysis center. He simply had to leave his room and walk down several corridors of the ship! Below are a couple of the companies we've come across that specialize in dialysis travel at sea:

Dialysis at Sea
www.DialysisatSea.com
Telephone in the United States and Canada: 1-800-544-7604
International: 01-101-727-518-7311

Dialysis on Demand Inc. Dialysis Dreams
www.dialysisdreams.com
Telephone: 1-954-527-3852

When in Doubt, Buy Insurance

A few years ago Daniel and Margie learned of a program, MedjetAssist, that provides them with some additional peace of mind while traveling. If you are younger than seventy-five years of age, for a fee you can become a MedjetAssist member. As a member, if you are hospitalized outside of a 150-mile radius of your home, MedjetAssist will fly you to a hospital of your choice at no charge in a medically equipped and staffed aircraft. For those who purchase this service, MedjetAssist essentially works as an insurance policy. Fortunately Daniel and Margie have never had to use their services, but it has given them a sense of comfort to know they have a quick exit strategy if a serious crisis were to occur far from the comfort of their home and their doctors.

Additional information on MedjetAssistance is available at

www.MedJetAssistance.com
info@madjetassistance.com
1-800-963-3538

While Daniel is optimistic about life and traveling, he is also realistic about the precarious nature of his health. For this reason, over the years if he and Margie are planning to take a big trip that involves a significant chunk of change, they will purchase travel insurance in advance. This way, if for some reason his or her health is compromised before they are scheduled to leave, they will only have to deal with the disappointment of missing out on the travel as opposed to the distress over losing money on airline tickets and hotel reservations that were left unused.

Think about Time Zones

Should you be traveling to or from home between dialysis sessions you may have to take into account time differences when calculating the time between sessions. For example, Daniel dialyzed on a Friday morning in Italy and was then scheduled to dialyze in Chicago on a Monday afternoon. Typically the longest Daniel would go between sessions was seventy-two hours. However, he realized Sunday night that it would be approximately eighty-six hours between sessions when the time change was accounted for. That same night he began feeling overly bloated and his breathing was becoming more labored. He called his home clinic and asked if he could move his dialysis earlier in the day on Monday. They were able to fit him in. Now he has learned that if he is in a similar situation in the future he will request an earlier session in advance.

Navigate the Language Divide

You may be worried about traveling to a country where you don't speak the language. Daniel has found that when he has traveled to another country there is always at least one person at the clinic who speaks English fairly well. That person informally becomes his ambassador at the clinic. To date, language has never been a problem for Margie or Daniel. If you are concerned, you may want to find someone at home or in your country of destination who can translate well. In the worst-case scenario, you can then pick up the phone and call your designated translator for some quick assistance.

What to Know for Transit: Carry Your Medical History, Medications, and Supplies

Daniel has learned to take his documented complete medical history with him whenever he travels. In the event that he needs to visit a hospital he can easily hand the physicians his medical profile. This document lists the following:

- Dates and durations of any past illnesses, surgeries, or fractures
- Current prescriptions and over-the-counter medications he is taking and their dosages
- Any allergies he has
- Names and telephone numbers of his dialysis clinic, his nephrologist, and all other specialists
- Parental medical history

The benefit of having this information typed up and on hand is that in the heat of a possibly stressful situation he and Margie do not have to rely on their ability to accurately recall all the pertinent details. They can instead rely on their "cheat sheet" to give the doctors a quick and accurate profile that can be used to provide the best possible care. It is not common that they've had to use this information when traveling.

In addition to these medical records, Daniel and Margie always pack the following supplies as a "just-in-case" measure should the access not coagulate:

- Scissors
- Gauze pads
- Tape
- Band-Aids
- Cortisporin or Bacitracin
- Latex gloves
- Thermometer

Daniel and Margie always carry their medications with them, including extra medications should their trip be extended for some unforeseen reason. At the time of writing this book, security measures taken by major airlines were subject to change in response to the ongoing level of threat of terrorism. While we'd advise you to carry all critical medical equipment, medication, and medical documents onboard and with you at all times, we recommend that you find out the latest rules and regulations regarding carry-on items. By the time you are reading this, they may have changed or they may require you to gather specific documentation in advance.

As mentioned earlier artificial erythropoietin helps dialysis patients ward off anemia. In the United States, this is an expensive drug, which is covered by Medicare. Outside of the United States it is not included in the cost of the treatment. If you plan to travel abroad you will need to purchase the drug in advance and carry it with you. In addition, it will need to be kept refrigerated. A black market exists for this medication. On the cruise, Daniel was told not to leave it in the refrigerator in his state room. Instead, the clinic asked him to bring it to them where they kept it refrigerated and under lock and key. When you are flying, you should pack the medication in a small insulated sack with ice or an icepack. If you have a long plane ride you may ask the stewardess for fresh ice midway through the flight. When Daniel and Margie arrive at the clinic for his first session, they bring his medicine with them and simply ask the staff to store it there for the duration of his stay. When he has the final session at that clinic he takes whatever medication remains home or to his next destination.

What to Know When You Arrive: Be Responsible for Your Care

On occasion Daniel and Margie have encountered scheduling mix-ups. For example, they have been given the wrong address for the clinic or the incorrect dialysis time. This is why it is critical whenever you arrive in your new destination to call the center to confirm the address and the treatment schedule. Also, before leaving for a trip, Daniel receives copies of the records of his last three treatments. He carries these with him and gives them to the head nurse when he enters the new clinic. The staff can then see how his recent treatments have gone, and this helps them to set up for the session. As he mentioned earlier, Daniel has learned on arriving at a new clinic always to tell the staff his dry weight, his blood pressure, how long he typically dialyzes, and the speed at which he dialyzes.

Account for Time

The longest that Daniel and Margie have ever traveled at one time was three weeks. However, if you are planning to travel longer you should arrange to have your blood chemistry checked at some point while you are on the road. This is important to ensure that you are still receiving the right dialysis prescription, as your chemistry may fluctuate over time.

What to Know When Staying Put: Plan for Emergencies

Travel in itself implies a visit to the unknown, someplace new. Truthfully, any adventure may result in the unexpected. In fact, even if you stay home, an adventure, usually the unwelcome kind, may actually come to you. Severe weather or a disaster may put you in a situation where you need to think on your feet. Extreme situations may make self-dialysis or travel anywhere, even to your regular center, impossible. Being prepared for such a situation will help minimize your worries, stay calm, and—in the event of a real emergency—keep you healthier until you can resume your normal treatment. To this end, the Centers for Medicare and Medicaid Services have created "Preparing for Emergencies: A Guide for People on Dialysis." The guide includes information on what to do in an emergency; travel tips; steps to prepare for an emergency, including an emergency food and supplies list and an emergency diet plan for three days; how to disinfect water; and how to get off a machine during an emergency evacuation. We certainly hope you never have such an adventure reach your doorstep, but if it does, you now know of an excellent resource that can help you prepare. You can request a free copy of this useful booklet at the address below:

1-800-Medicare
Centers for Medicare and Medicaid Services
7500 Security Boulevard
Baltimore, MD 21244-1850
www.Medicare.gov

And should you be very worried about the threat of a disaster and managing dialysis in its midst you will be comforted to hear that when Hurricane Katrina hit the Gulf Coast in 2005, every single one of the dialysis patients was successfully triaged and cared for at alternative centers. We spoke with the director of the largest dialysis center in Houston who explained to us that many dialysis centers surrounding the areas damaged by the storm provided around-the-clock care. If needed, centers would have shifts in the middle of the night. Initially, some individuals had to wait a day or two longer than usual to receive care, but ultimately everyone was accounted for and all those who were uprooted found temporary or permanent new clinics to call home.

All Systems Go

Whether you are contemplating emergency preparedness or your dream vacation, life as a dialysis patient very much revolves around planning. Now it is time to make a plan. If you never cared in the least bit for travel before you went on dialysis, we don't expect you to put down this book and immediately call your travel agent. But if you have an adventurous soul or a yen for travel, then just because a piece of your body doesn't work properly doesn't mean you have to stifle your desires to meet new people and see new sights. And if you are on hemodialysis, you now have the opportunity to have a bird's-eye view into a world that most tourists never see! You can meet and speak to people at your destination clinics that you never would have met. Most run-of-the-mill tourists don't have such a sure-fire way to meet locals, but you have an automatic entrée to the natives. Regardless of whether you do self-dialysis or in-center dialysis, travel is a wonderful, healthy form of escapism and even though your baggage (literally and figuratively) will follow you wherever you go, you can lighten your load by taking the leap.

Afterword

A ND SO WE arrive at the end of the book with a few parting thoughts we'd like to share. As we mentioned earlier, according to the National Kidney Foundation one out of every nine people in the United States is affected by kidney disease. This statistic does not mean that these affected individuals will all eventually be on dialysis, but it does mean that kidney disease is not nearly as rare as most people think. And although this book is not preventive in nature and we are primarily addressing many individuals who already find themselves on dialysis, we would like to do our part to influence the family members of dialysis patients and anyone who is not already on dialysis to periodically have their GFR levels checked as a measurement of their kidney function. We would encourage everyone to know their GFR levels and to take their physician's recommended steps to prevent a significant decline of kidney function. In many cases, if caught early enough, renal failure can be prevented or at the very least slowed. Ideally, some day the rates of individuals undergoing dialysis annually will be on the decline instead of the rise and the audience for a book like this will diminish in size.

For those individuals who are already on dialysis, we commend you for what you do to stay alive. We know that it is not easy. You endure much. But we also know that, like ours, your families and loved ones are very appreciative of the many moments, conversations, and memories shared with you that they might otherwise not have had. If knowing that is sometimes not enough to bolster your resolve, you may have to rely on special occasions to keep you on track and motivated to put up with dialysis. And what it takes to get you to those milestones or celebrations will certainly take a backseat to the joy of the moment.

Appendix A

Glossary of Terms

Access—General term used to describe the site where the blood will enter and exit your body during hemodialysis. Also commonly referred to as "lifeline." Temporary accesses are typically used short term whereas permanent accesses are used long term.

Arteriovenous (AV) fistula—A type of permanent access used for hemodialysis surgically created by attaching a vein directly to an artery.

Arteriovenous (AV) graft—A type of permanent access used for hemodialysis surgically created by attaching an artery indirectly to a vein using a small plastic tube.

Anemia—A decrease in the amount of red blood cells that are needed to carry enough oxygen to meet the body's needs. Healthy kidneys produce the hormones needed to create red blood cells. Chronic kidney failure can cause anemia. Symptoms of anemia include lethargy, lack of appetite, and shortness of breath.

Blood urea nitrogen (BUN)—A measure of the waste product of protein metabolism. Its removal is a marker of the efficiency of dialysis.

Calcium—A mineral that is important for strong bones.

Catheter—A flexible hollow tube that is inserted into and juts out from the patient's body. Catheters are sometimes used as temporary accesses for hemodialysis and are the main conduit for PD exchanges to the abdomen.

Chronic kidney disease—The term used to generically describe conditions that damage your kidneys and decrease their ability to function properly.

Chronic renal failure—Condition in which the kidneys fail permanently. The nonworking kidneys cannot function again as in acute renal failure, which can be reversed.

Continuous ambulatory peritoneal dialysis (CAPD)—A form of peritoneal dialysis that involves several manual exchanges daily. No machine is used.

Continuous cycling peritoneal dialysis (CCPD)—A form of peritoneal dialysis that involves continuous mechanized exchanges nightly and a possible manual exchange daily. Also sometimes referred to as ambulatory peritoneal dialysis (APD).

Creatinine—A substance produced by the muscles and used to detect kidney failure.

Cycler—The machine that is used to mechanically perform CCPD exchanges overnight.

Diabetes—A condition characterized by high blood sugar resulting from the body's inability to use sugar efficiently. Diabetes can cause kidney failure.

Dialysate—The cleansing solution that is used in the dialyzer or in the peritoneum to remove the excess fluid and toxins from the blood. This special mixture of chemicals and water allows for the removal of certain chemicals from the blood and addition of certain chemicals to the blood.

Dialysis—The process of cleaning wastes from the blood artificially.

Dialyzer—A part of the hemodialysis machine that acts as an artificial kidney removing excess fluids and toxins from the blood.

Edema—Swelling caused by an excess buildup of fluids in the body.

End-stage renal disease (ESRD)—A term often used by the medical industry to signify diminished kidney function to the point that an individual must either receive dialysis or a transplant in order to live.

Endocrinologist—A physician who specializes in the care and treatment of the endocrine system, which is the body's system of glands and hormones.

Epogen (EPO)—A man-made pharmaceutical substitute for erythropoietin.

Erythropoietin—A hormone that healthy kidneys create that signals the production of red blood cells. It is now artificially manufactured by the pharmaceutical industry under several trademarked names.

Exchange—The process of peritoneal dialysis consisting of the fill, the dwell, and the drain. First the abdomen is filled with fluid, the abdomen retains the fluid for a period of time, and the abdomen is drained of fluid. The complete process is called an exchange.

Glomerular filtration rate (GFR)—A measurement that determines the health of a kidney. Measured as a percentage, the estimated GFR is the amount of kidney functionality that remains. A GFR of 15% or less means that a person requires dialysis or transplantation to live.

Glomerulonephritis—A disease resulting from an inflammation of the kidney that destroys kidney tissue.

Hemodialysis—A treatment process that removes the blood from the body and cleanses it of excess fluids and impurities using a filter called a dialyzer.

Hypertension—A disorder in which blood pressure remains abnormally high.

Immunosuppressant—Drugs given to suppress the natural responses of the body's immune system. They are given to people with transplants to prevent organ rejection.

Iron—A mineral found in bone marrow necessary for the production of hemoglobin, the oxygen-carrying component in red blood cells. Eating iron-rich foods and taking iron supplements can help prevent anemia.

Kidneys—A pair of organs located near the middle of the back that filter and remove excess fluid and toxic impurities from the blood, produce hormones needed to control blood pressure and create red blood cells, and balance the level of minerals and chemicals in the body such as sodium, potassium, calcium, and phosphorus.

Living nonrelated donor—An individual who is willing to donate a kidney but is not related by blood to the patient in need.

Living related donor—An individual who is willing to donate a kidney and is related to the person needing it.

Modality—Form of treatment. Different forms of treatment for nonfunctioning kidneys include transplantation, hemodialysis, and peritoneal dialysis.

Nephrologist: A physician who specializes in the care and study of kidneys, their function, and the diseases associated with them.

Peritoneal cavity: The space in the abdomen that, in peritoneal dialysis, contains the diasylate and removes unhealthy toxins and fluids from the blood.

Peritoneal dialysis (PD): A type of dialysis that uses the peritoneal cavity and dialysate to cleanse the blood of impurities and excess fluid without removing it from the body.

Peritoneal membrane—The lining of the abdominal cavity resembling cellophane with tiny holes that is used to sift out excess fluids and harmful toxins during an exchange.

Peritonitis—An infection of the abdomen sometimes associated with peritoneal dialysis.

Phosphorus—A substance found in many of the foods that we eat. Healthy kidneys work to monitor the balance of phosphorus levels in the body so that they are neither too low nor too high. Too much phosphorus can cause calcium to be removed from your bones, which weakens them.

Phosphorus binders—Medications that prevent phosphorus we eat from being absorbed into the blood.

Polycystic kidney disease—An inherited disease characterized by the buildup of cysts on the kidneys that destroy kidney tissue and can cause kidney failure.

Potassium—A mineral in your blood that helps your heart and muscles work properly. Healthy kidneys work to balance potassium levels in the body so that they are neither too low nor too high.

Renal—Relating to the kidneys.

Reuse—A procedure in hemodialysis in which the dialyzer is cleaned and tested after each session before being reused by the same patient for the next session. The clean dialyzer is reused with the same person only.

Transplantation—The surgical procedure of placing a kidney from a donor into a recipient. There are three types of donations: cadaver, living-related, and living nonrelated.

Ultrafiltration rate—The rate at which liquid and impurities move out of the bloodstream during hemodialysis.

Urea—A waste product that the body makes when protein is broken down. The rate of urea removal from the blood by dialysis is a measure of how the dialysis treatment is working.

Uremia—The condition when waste products that are normally removed by the kidneys build up in the blood, leading to symptoms such as poor appetite, nausea, vomiting, itching, fatigue, and confusion.

Urine—Liquid waste product filtered from the blood by the kidneys.

Urologist—A surgeon who specializes in the diagnosis and treatment of diseases of the urinary tract and urogenital system.

Vascular surgeon—A surgeon who specializes in the diagnosis and treatment of disorders of arteries and veins. This physician performs the operation to create an access.

Appendix B

Helpful Resources

Listed below are just a handful of the resources currently available to aid renal care patients and their family members. These are the resources that we've found to be particularly helpful and will likely be a good starting point for you as you seek out additional information.

General Educational Resources

American Association of Kidney Patients (AAKP)
3505 E. Frontage Rd., Ste. 315
Tampa, FL 33607-1796
1-800-749-2257
www.aakp.org

AAKP has twelve chapters nationwide and 12,000 members. This organization has a wealth of materials including newsletters, booklets, brochures, and magazines available on all topics pertaining to kidney disease.

Davita Patient Citizens
www.dialysispatients.org

Educational website sponsored by DaVita Inc., the largest independent provider of dialysis centers in the United States.

End Stage Renal Disease Networks
Eighteen regional networks each covering a different part of the United States. To receive information about your regional network contact:

1527 Huguenot Road
Midlothian, Virginia 23113
1-804-794-2586
www.esrdnetworks.org

These networks were created to act as the liaison between the federal Health Care Finance Administration and the providers of dialysis and transplantation services. Each network provides patient services and education.

Home Dialysis Central
www.homedialysis.org

This website includes descriptions of existing types of peritoneal and home hemodialysis, success stories, discussion boards, listings of centers that offer home dialysis, information on pending legislation, updates on new home dialysis technology, and Medicare reimbursement information.

Kidney Options
www.kidneyoptions.com

Educational website sponsored by Fresenius Medical Care North America. Fresenius Medical Care is the world's largest provider of dialysis products and services.

Kidney School
www.kidneyschool.org

Interactive web-based learning program in twenty-minute modules designed to help educate kidney patients so that they can take a more active role in their health care.

Life Options
c/o Medical Education Institute, Inc.
414 D'Onofrio Drive Suite 200
Madison, WI 53719
1-800-468-7777
www.lifeoptions.org

This organization has developed an abundance of useful materials on how to live well with kidney disease.

The National Kidney Foundation (NKF)
30 East 33rd Street
New York, NY 10016
1-800-622-9010
www.kidney.org

NKF has a wealth of materials including newsletters, booklets, brochures, and magazines available on all topics pertaining to kidney disease.

The National Alliance for Caregiving (NAC)
4720 Montgomery Lane, 5th Floor
Bethesda, MD 20814
www.caregiving.org
The NAC is a nonprofit coalition of national organizations focusing on issues of family caregiving. The organization has publications, tips, and guides for caregivers.

The Organ Procurement and Transplantation Network (OPTN)
www.optn.org
A real-time UNOS (see below) run website which provides OPTN data including organ procurement waitlists and to-date transplants in the United States.

Transplant Living
www.transplantliving.org
A website operated by the United Network for Organ Sharing (UNOS) that provides transplant information, resources, and tools for patients, families, and friends.

United Network for Organ Sharing (UNOS)
Post Office Box 2484
Richmond, Virginia 23218
1-888-894-6361
www.unos.org
A nonprofit, scientific, and educational organization that administers the Organ Procurement and Transplantation Network, a unified network linking all professionals involved in organ transplantation; facilitates organ matching and donation; collects data about every transplant occurring in the United States; and works to develop organ donation and transplantation policies.

Travel Resources

Dialysis at Sea
13555 Automobile Blvd, Suite 220
Clearwater, FL 33762
1-800-544-7604
www.dialysisatsea.com
The largest worldwide provider of dialysis services aboard cruise ships.

Dialysis on Demand Inc.
3200 So. Andrews Ave., Suite #115
Ft. Lauderdale, FL. 33316-4122
1-954-527-3852
www.dialysisdreams.com

Company specializing in dialysis cruises.

Easter Seals Project Action
1425 K Street, NW, Suite 200
Washington, DC 20005
1-800-659-6428
TTD for hearing impaired: 202-347-7385
www.projectaction.org

Can provide a list of accessible transportation services in the United States for people with disabilities.

Global Dialysis
www.globaldialysis.com

A website created to aid dialysis travelers in locating dialysis centers around the globe. Includes a database of centers as well as resources and information pertaining to dialysis and travel.

MedjetAssistance
Birmingham International Airport
4900 69th Street North
Birmingham, Alabama 35206
1-800-963-3538
www.medjetassistance.com

Provider of annual membership plans, similar to an insurance plan, that would cover the costs of an emergency medical evacuation from anywhere in the world to a hospital of your choice.

Professional and Financial Resources

ADA & IT Technical Assistance Centers
For your local center call or visit the web at
1-800-949-4232
www.adata.org

Provides information about the network of Disability Business Technical Assistance Centers (DBTACs) throughout the United States that exist for the use of individuals covered under the Americans with Disabilities Act. These centers provide a variety of training, technical, advisory, and educational services.

American Kidney Fund
www.kidneyfund.org
1-800-638-8299
The leading source of direct financial aid to chronic kidney disease patients in the United States.

Centers for Medicare and Medicaid Services
7500 Security Boulevard Baltimore, MD 21244
Toll-Free: 1-877-267-232
www.cms.hhs.gov
Information pertaining to both Medicare and Medicaid services. However, if you have inquiries specifically about Medicare you should start at the Medicare-specific website and 1-800-MEDICARE number listed below.

Kidney Drug Coverage
Kidney Medicare Drugs Awareness and Education Initiative
c/o National Kidney Foundation
30 East 33rd Street
New York, NY 10016
1-800-622-9010
www.kidneydrugcoverage.org
This initiative was created to provide timely, reliable, and up-to-date information about Medicare drug coverage for kidney patients.

Medicare
1-800-MEDICARE (1-800-633-4227)
www.Medicare.gov
The official U.S. government site for people with Medicare. Information, resources, and tools pertaining to Medicare.

Partnership for Prescription Assistance
1-888-4PPA-NOW (1-888-477-2669)
www.pparx.org
A collaboration of companies, health care providers, and organizations to provide low-cost or no-cost prescription drugs to patients in need. Contact them to learn more about which programs you may qualify for.

RxAssist

www.rxassist.org

A comprehensive web directory of patient assistance programs run by pharmaceutical companies to provide low-cost or no-cost medications to patients in need.

United States Department of Labor Employee Benefits Security Administration
Frances Perkins Building
200 Constitution Avenue, NW
Washington, DC 20210
1-866-444-3272
TTY: 1-877-889-5627
www.dol.gov/ebsa

This government entity can provide you with a great deal of information regarding health care plans, benefits, and rights under the Health Insurance Portability and Accountability Act (HIPAA) and the Consolidated Omnibus Budget Reconciliation Act (COBRA).

United States Social Security Administration
Office of Public Inquiries
Windsor Park Building
6401 Security Blvd.
Baltimore, MD 21235
Toll Free: 1-800-772-1213
TTY: 1-800-325-0778
www.socialsecurity.gov

Can provide information on Social Security Disability Insurance and Supplemental Security Income. Can also refer you to your State Vocational Rehabilitation office. For an online listing of these offices visit www.jan.wvu.edu/sbses/vocrehab.htm

United States Social Security Administration—The Work Site
www.ssa.gov/work

The website provides basic information about the Ticket to Work program that was designed to help individuals who are receiving Social Security Disability benefits return to work. For additional information about the Ticket to Work program visit www.yourtickettowork.com or call 1-866-968-7842.

Legal Resources

Equal Employment Opportunity Commission
U.S. Equal Employment Opportunity Commission
P.O. Box 7033
Lawrence, Kansas 66044
Toll Free: 1-800-669-4000
TTY for hearing impaired: 1-800-669-6820
www.eeoc.gov
Can help individuals with facts and guidance related to antidiscrimination laws, disability rights, and steps to file charges of discrimination.

Patient Advocate Foundation
1-800-532-5774
www.patientadvocate.org
A national nonprofit organization that assists with mediation and advocacy when a patient's fair rights to care, financial support, or employment are denied.

Books

Chronic Hemodialysis as a Way of Life
J.W. Czaczkes, Ph.D., M.D., and A. Kaplan De-Nour, M.D.
Brunner/Mazel Inc. 1978

Chronically Happy: Joyful Living in Spite of Chronic Illness
Lori Hartwell
Poetic Media Press, 2002

Cooking for David: A Culinary Dialysis Cookbook
Sara Coleman and Dorothy Gordon
Culinary Kidney Cooks; Spiral edition (July 2000)
www.culinarykidneycooks.com

Dialysis: An Unanticipated Journey. A Life Experience on Dialysis for 30+ Years
David L. Axtmann
Tucky Paws Publishing, 2001

Eating Well, Living Well with Kidney Disease:
Dietary Approaches to Healthy Living from the Sarah W. Stedman Center for Nutritional Studies at Duke University Medical Center
Steve J. Schwab, M.D., and Dorothy W. Bartholomay, M.P.H., R.D.
Penguin Group, 1997

Heroes: 100 Stories of Living with Kidney Failure
Devon Philips, Editor
Grosvenor House Press Inc., 1998

Kidney Failure: The Facts
Stewart Cameron
Oxford University Press, 1996

When Your Kidneys Fail
Mickie Hall Faris, M.P.H., M.B.A.
National Kidney Foundation of Southern California, 1994

Journals, Magazines, and Newsletters

aakpRENALIFE
A publication of the American Association of Kidney Patients
info@aakp.org
1-800-749-2257

Published every other month; features a range of educational information for renal patients.

Dialysis & Transplantation
Wiley Periodicals Inc.
www.interscience.wiley.com
1-201-748-5764

A monthly journal written for medical professionals in the field of renal care. A bit more medical and technical than other resources listed here. But if you happen to be a medical professional on dialysis you may find some of the articles very interesting.

Family Focus
1-800-622-9010
www.kidney.org

A Publication of the National Kidney Foundation
Published quarterly. Includes excellent stories, anecdotes, and helpful information for renal care patients on all topics relevant to living with chronic kidney disease.

Kidney Beginnings: The Magazine
A Publication of the American Association of Kidney Patients
info@aakp.org
1-800-749-2257

Published quarterly; includes articles, news items, and features of interest to those at risk or recently diagnosed with kidney disease.

Notes

Preface

1. Axtmann, *Dialysis An Unanticipated Journey*, 17.

Chapter One

1. National Kidney Foundation, www.kidney.org, "20 million Americans—1 in 9 US adults—have CKD and another 20 million more are at increased risk. . . . Nearly half of people with an advanced form of kidney disease do not know they have weak or failing kidneys, according to recent research published in the *American Journal of Kidney Diseases*, the official journal of the National Kidney Foundation."

2. Lopresi, "At the Olympics, a Father's Love Knows No Limits," www.usatoday.com, August 20, 2004.

Chapter Three

1. Department of Health and Human Services, National Institutes of Health, National Institute of Diabetes and Digestive and Kidney Diseases, Division of Kidney Urologic and Hematologic Diseases. *United States Renal Data System 2005 Annual Data Report: Atlas of End-Stage Renal Disease in the United States*, 97.

Chapter Four

1. The Organ Procurement and Transplantation Network. www.optn.org, Kidney Kaplan-Meier Graft Survival Rates for Transplants Performed: 1997–2004. Search National Data, Survival, Kidney, Graft, by Age.

2. The Organ Procurement and Transplantation Network. www.optn.org, Kidney Kaplan-Meier Graft Survival Rates for Transplants Performed: 1997–2004. Search National Data, Survival, Kidney, Graft, by Age.

3. The Organ Procurement and Transplantation Network. www.optn.org, Kidney Kaplan-Meier Graft Survival Rates for Transplants Performed: January 1, 1988—August, 31 2006. Search National Data, Transplant, Kidney, by Age.

4. Department of Health and Human Services, National Institutes of Health, National Institute of Diabetes and Digestive and Kidney Diseases, Division of Kidney Urologic and Hematologic Diseases. *United States Renal Data System 2005 Annual Data Report: Atlas of End-Stage Renal Disease in the United States,* 100, 4.d.

5. Department of Health and Human Services, National Institutes of Health, National Institute of Diabetes and Digestive and Kidney Diseases, Division of Kidney Urologic and Hematologic Diseases. *United States Renal Data System 2005 Annual Data Report: Atlas of End-Stage Renal Disease in the United States,* "One-year patient and graft survival rates have improved in the past eight years . . . ," 150.

6. The Organ Procurement and Transplantation Network. www.optn.org, Kidney Kaplan-Meier Graft Survival Rates for Transplants Performed: January 1, 1988—August 31, 2006. Search National Data, Transplant, Kidney, by Donor Type.

7. The Organ Procurement and Transplantation Network. www.optn.org, Waiting List Candidates as of Today.

8. The Organ Procurement and Transplantation Network. www.optn.org, Kidney Kaplan-Meier Graft Survival Rates for Transplants Performed: January 1, 1988—August, 31 2006. Search National Data, Transplant, Kidney, by Donor Type.

Chapter Six

1. Riis, J., et al. "Ignorance of Hedonic Adaptation to Hemodialysis: A Study Using Ecological Momentary Assessment," 3–9.

2. Watnick S., P. Kirwin., R. Mahnensmith, et al., "The Prevalence and Treatment of Depression among Patients Starting Dialysis," 105–110.

Guzman, S. J., and Nicassio, P. M., "The Contribution of Negative and Positive Illness Schemas to Depression in Patients with End-Stage Renal Disease," 517–534.

Chapter Eight

1. United States Department of Justice Civil Rights Division, *A Guide to Disability Rights Laws,* 1.

2. United States Department of Labor. www.dol.gov/esa, Compliance Assistance—Family Medical Leave Act (FMLA).

Bibliography

Ahlstrom, Timothy P. *The Kidney Patient's Book: New Treatment, New Hope.* Delran, N.J.: Great Issues Press, 1991.

The American Association of Kidney Patients. *AAKP Patient Plan Phase 1: Diagnosis to Treatment Choice.* Tampa: AAKP, n.d.

The American Association of Kidney Patients. *The Iron Story.* Tampa: AAKP, 2002.

The American Association of Kidney Patients. *Patient to Patient: A Newsletter Series for the AAKP Patient Plan,* 1(1). Tampa: AAKP, 1999.

The American Association of Kidney Patients. *Understanding Your Hemodialysis Options.* Tampa: AAKP, n.d.

Axtmann, David L. *Dialysis: An Unanticipated Journey. A Life Experience on Dialysis for 30+ Years.* Cottage Grove, Minn.: Tucky Paws Publishing, 2001.

Boccanfuso, Judy, RD, CSR, and Michelle Yamanoha, MS, RD. *Making the Best Choices for Holiday Eating.* Daly City, Calif.: Council on Renal Nutrition Northern California/Northern Nevada, n.d.

Brassil, Donna F., RN, MA, CURN, and Jean H. Lewis, BSN, RN, CNP. "Sexuality and the Renal Patient." *Kidney Beginnings: The Magazine,* 2 (2) (June/July 2003).

Brown, Wendy W., MD, and Bobbie Knotek, RN, BSN. "Do You Have Questions about Kidney Failure and Your Sex Life?" *Family Focus: A Publication of the National Kidney Foundation,* 13 (2) (Spring 2004).

Cameron, Stewart. *Kidney Failure: The Facts.* New York: Oxford University Press, 1981.

Church & Dwight Co., Inc. *A Guide to Taking Control of Your Life on Dialysis: Helpful Information for Hemodialysis Patients.* Princeton, N.J.: Church & Dwight, 2001.

Czaczkes, J.W., PhD, MD, and A. Kaplan De-Nour, MD. *Chronic Hemodialysis as a Way of Life.* New York: Brunner/Mazel, 1978.

Department of Health and Human Services, National Institutes of Health, National Institute of Diabetes and Digestive and Kidney Diseases, Division of

Kidney Urologic and Hematologic Diseases. *United States Renal Data System 2005 Annual Data Report: Atlas of End-Stage Renal Disease in the United States.* Minneapolis: Minneapolis Medical Research Foundation, 2005.

"Doctors Fall Short on Kidney Care, Survey Shows." *New York Times,* August 8, 2006.

Gahagan, Jayne D. *Dialysis and You: A Self-Help Guide for Patients.* Evanston, Ill.: J. D. Gahagan, Interpretive Writing Service, Inc. 1977.

Guzman, S. J., and P. M. Nicassio. "The Contribution of Negative and Positive Illness Schemas to Depression in Patients with End-Stage Renal Disease." *Journal of Behavioral Medicine* 6 (December 26, 2003): 517–534.

Hall Faris, Mickie, MPH, MBA. *When Your Kidneys Fail: The Easy-to-Use Resource for People with Kidney Disease.* 3rd ed. Ed. Carol J. Amato. Los Angeles: National Kidney Foundation of Southern California, 1994.

Hartwell, Lori. *Chronically Happy: Joyful Living in Spite of Chronic Illness.* San Francisco: Poetic Media Press, 2002.

Hema Metrics. *Using the Crit-Line Monitor to Manage Your Dry Weight for an Optimal Hemodialysis Treatment.* Kaysville, Utah: Hema Metrics, 2003.

"Kidney Transplants from Live Donors Increase." *Chicago Tribune,* December 5, 2004.

Lopresi, Mike. "At the Olympics, a Father's Love Knows No Limits." www.usatoday.com, August 20, 2004.

National Kidney Foundation. www.kidney.org/atoz. "A to Z Health Guide: Your Comprehensive Guide to Kidney Disease and Related Conditions." February 2007.

National Kidney Foundation. *About Chronic Kidney Disease: A Guide for Patients and Their Families.* New York: NKF, 2002.

National Kidney Foundation. *Dining Out with Confidence.* New York: NKF, 2004.

National Kidney Foundation. *Family Focus.* Patient Advocacy, 14 (1) (Winter 2005).

National Kidney Foundation. *Family Focus.* Mental Health, 14 (3) (Summer 2005).

National Kidney Foundation. *Health Care Team Facts: Social Work Services for the Person with Kidney Failure.* New York: NKF, 1998.

National Kidney Foundation. *Getting the Most from Your Treatment: What You Need to Know about Your Access.* New York: NKF, 1998.

National Kidney Foundation. *Taking Control: Money Matters for People with Chronic Kidney Disease.* New York: National Endowment for Financial Education, 2005.

National Kidney Foundation of Northern California/Northern Nevada. Happy Holidays: Festive Foods, Family and Friends. Foster City, Calif.: National Kidney Foundation of Northern California/Northern Nevada, n.d.

National Kidney Foundation, www.kidney.org. Lists facts about chronic kidney disease including: 20 million Americans—1 in 9 US adults—have CKD.

"Next Generation: Do-It-Yourself Dialysis." *University of Chicago Magazine*, October, 2004.

Nagourney, Eric. "Health and Happiness Aren't Always Linked." Science Times, *New York Times*, February 15, 2005.

The Organ Procurement and Transplantation Network. www.optn.org. This website contains data on the graft survival rates of transplanted kidneys. Data are revised over time.

Phillips, Devon, ed. *Heroes: 100 Stories of Living with Kidney Failure.* Montreal, Quebec: Grosvenor House Press, 1998.

Phillips, Robert H., PhD. *Coping with Kidney Failure: A Guide to Living with Kidney Failure for You and Your Family.* Wayne, N.J.: Avery Publishing Group, 1987.

www.quotedb.com. An online database of quotations, including the quotation on travel by St. Augustine.

The Renal Network Inc. *Your Lifeline: Access Care.* Indianapolis, Ind.: Renal Network, 2000.

Renshaw, Domeena C., MD. "Sexuality and Renal Patients." *Medical Sex Journal* 4(2) (1993): 34–42.

Riis, J., G. Lowenstein, J. Baron, C. Jepson, A. Fagerlin, and P. A. Ubel. "Ignorance of Hedonic Adaptation to Hemodialysis: A Study Using Ecological Momentary Assessment." *Journal of Experimental Psychology: General* 134 (1) (2005): 3–9.

Schwab, Steve J., MD, and Dorothy W. Bartholomay, MPH, RD. *Eating Well Living Well with Kidney Disease: Dietary Approaches to Healthy Living.* New York: Penguin Books, 1997.

Shaft, Laurie, RD, and Gambro Healthcare. *Happy Holidays: Holiday Eating Tips.* Daly City, California: National Kidney Foundation of Northern California and Council on Renal Nutrition of Northern California/Northern Nevada, 1999.

Tracy, Kathleen. *Willem Kolff and the Invention of the Dialysis Machine.* Bear, Delaware: Mitchell Lane Publishers, 2002.

United Network for Organ Sharing. *What Every Patient Needs to Know.* Richmond, Virginia: UNOS, 2002.

United States Department of Justice Civil Rights Division. *A Guide to Disability Rights Laws.* September, 2005.

United States Department of Labor. www.dol.gov/esa. Compliance Assistance–Family Medical Leave Act (FMLA.)

Watnick, S., P. Kirwin, R. Mahnensmith, et al. "The Prevalence and Treatment of Depression among Patients Starting Dialysis." *American Journal of Kidney Disease,* 41(1): 105–110, 2003.

Index